PERIOPERATIVE LASER NURSING

A Practical Guide

Carolyn J. MacKety, RN, MA

Laser Centers of America

Laser Centers of America
1111 St. Gregory Street
Cincinnati, Ohio 45202

Perioperative Laser Nursing
A Practical Guide
Second Edition

Library of Congress Catalog Card Number 83-51728

Copyright© 1989 by Laser Centers of America, 1111 St. Gregory Street, Cincinnati, Ohio 45202.
All rights reserved. No part of this book may be reproduced, stored in a retrieval system or transmitted in any form or by any means, electronic, mechanical, photocopying, recording or otherwise, without written permission from the publisher, except for brief quotations embodied in critical articles and reviews.

Printed in the United States of America

ISBN: 0-943432-21-9

LASER PRAYER

God, our Creator, at the beginning of time You gave us the gift of light and through the ages You have shared with us Your Spirit of Wisdom to help us better understand this precious gift and its many potential uses.

From the discovery of candles, to refracted light to electric sources of light and now, in our day, Laser light, You have helped us to use this gift of creation for the betterment of the human family.

We ask You bless this new endeavor so that our efforts may bring healing to Your people and honor and glory to Your name. We ask this of You, our God who lives and reigns now and forever.

This prayer was given at the dedication of the Pittsburgh Laser Center at St. Francis Hospital, Pittsburgh Pennsylvania by Father John and used for the dedication of this book by his permission.

DEDICATION

During the advancement of a very exciting nursing career, moving out of clinical practice in the operating room, to administrative nursing responsibilities, and becoming a nurse entrepreneur; many persons have touched my life to make my "impossible dreams" come true.

First, I'd like to thank a wonderful supportive family, parents who have stood-by, my brother, Jerry who's my dearest friend, and my children Dan, Dave, Steve, and Laura, who gave me reason to "reach for the stars!" Friends from every walks of life, too many to mention; who have always supported my efforts.

My "launch " into lasers happened in 1981, and I must "reach-out" and recognize special people who where there and part of a real team effort. There are: Drs. Jim McCaughan, Jack Lomano, Toni Neri and Jim Andrews (who recently died). Others are Greg who "turned-me-on" to lasers, Benjamin Holland; who was my mentor and gave me the opportunity to reach my potential as an administrator, Violet Mc Donnogh, friend and former secretary, who struggled with me through the first edition of this book, the O.R. Recovery, Ambulatory Surgery Staffs, the Laser Team and lastly a friend, always there, never questioning, always supportive Kay Martin.

During the last five years, the people in the laser field, both industrial and medical have had a significant influence in the development of my career. Their support to advance nurses " knowledge and ability" to work with lasers have been tremendous. I've been privileged to develop very special friendships, and I love each of you!

To those clients who trusted me to inform and help them in the development of their laser programs. Thank you for your confidence.

To my former associate, Carol Wirth, who adopted my baby, Laser Consultants Inc., I wish a wonderful future. To my associates at Laser Centers of America and especially Dr. Stephen Joffe, M.D. my boss, for the opportunity to broaden my horizons!

To all the nurses and laser support persons who have attended my workshops, seminars, and lectures, and to the nurses of the future I dedicate the book to each of you, and challenge you to stand-up and be counted for the future of nursing.

A special **Thank You** to; Michael Blakeslee, R.T., Medical Center Hospital of Vermont for taking the time to read and review this manuscript for interest and clarity of text.

CONTENTS

Preface	ix
History	xi - xii

Part 1 — 1 - 41
Technical Aspects of Lasers

Chapter 1 Basic Laser Biophysics	3 - 12
Chapter 2 Types of Lasers	13 - 18
Chapter 3 Tissue Effects of Lasers	19 - 24
Chapter 4 Laser Safety	25 - 41

Part 2 — 43 - 70
Laser Program Development

Chapter 5 How to Decide	45 - 51
Chapter 6 Procurement and Installation	52 - 61
Chapter 7 The Administrative Role	62 - 70

Part 3 — 71 - 135
Lasers in Medicine and Surger... The Nurses Role

Chapter 8 Clinical Applications of Lasers	73 - 79
Chapter 9 The Laser Team	80 - 84
Chapter 10 The Perioperative Laser Nurse	85 - 90

Chapter 11 Perioperative Patient Care	91 - 129
Section I Assessment	91 - 93
Section II Intraoperative Responsibilities	94 - 101
Section III Specific Procedural Information	101 - 128
Chapter 12 The Future . . .	130 - 135

Appendix   137 - 158

    Glossary   139 - 142
    Information for Patients   143 - 145
    Home Care Instructions   146 - 147
    Job Description   148 - 150
    Orientation for Nurses   151 - 152
    Reimbursement Form   153
    Classroom Requirements   154 - 155
    Selected Readings   156 - 157
    Laser Log   158

PREFACE

Caring for patients who have laser procedures is becoming an expanded nursing role, and affects our daily practice. The use of lasers in medicine and surgery is proliferating in areas, from medical and surgical to interventional applications.

Lasers have been used in Ophthalmology since 1962, however, only since 1972 have they moved into other areas of medicine. First, lasers were placed in operating rooms. Currently, lasers are being installed in ambulatory surgical suites, endoscopy suites, to include gastroenterology and pulmonary. Lasers are also being used in physician's offices and clinic areas. Soon lasers will be in radiology departments and various diagnostic laboratories. The scope of laser utilization in health care facilities are still in its infancy.

As nurses are the patients advocate during health care delivery, they must expand their knowledge base, to keep abreast of this fast paced technology. This book will help the nurse in expanding this knowledge base by supplying laser information in laser biophysics and their photobiological interaction in the pathophysiology of tissue. Other information that must be assimilated regarding lasers is; the safety concerns, maintenance of equipment, use of the laser accessories, and the laser support personnel responsibilities. To help nurses to make proper decisions regarding patient assessment and care plan development, there's significant information on the care of the patient perioperatively.

Resulting from the economic concerns of the health care delivery today, I'll try to address administrative responsibility, laser acquisition, laser economics and marketing techniques.

As laser technology's fast paced growth won't allow this book to stay current regarding the future applications, only limited information on future trends will be in a chapter.

When the reader completes the assimilation of this information they'd have a general knowledge of laser systems, safety, applications in the specialties currently using lasers, administrative concerns, economics, nursing responsibilities, and examine the future for our expanded role in the delivery of quality patient care.

HISTORY OF LASERS IN MEDICINE AND SURGERY

Light **A**mplification by the **S**imulated **E**mission of **R**adiation, is a theory first postulated by Albert Einstein in the early 1900's. He noted that light and color were the results of wave properties and interactions with photons. Like sunlight, radio-waves, and light produced by a 100 watt tungsten light bulb, a laser beam in electro-magnetic energy. Unlike X-ray or other ionizing radiation, lasers don't produce the dangerous effects of gamma radiation

Although the light theory was founded by Christian Hauggen (1642-1695), and the particle theory of light by Isaac Newton (1642-1727), Einstein's laser principles in medicine evolved about 1958.

In 1958, Drs. Schawlow and Townes, physicists at Standford University in California, developed the principle of Light Amplification by the Stimulated Emission of Radiation using microwaves. In 1960, Dr. Theodore Maiman, PhD. invented the ruby laser, but not used clinically until 1962. In 1961, Dr. Kumar Patel of Bell Laboratories in New Jersey researched gaseous lasers for communication. In 1963, at Standford University, Drs. M. Flocks and C. Zweny used the ruby laser for retina repairs because that wavelength of energy is absorbed primarily by blue pigmented material. By the mid-1960's the ruby laser had been replaced by an Argon-ion generated beam, an inert element that coagulates, but doesn't vaporize red tissue. In 1965, the Argon-ion laser was used in Ophthalmology in the treatment of Diabetic Retinopathy. In 1970, Drs Thomas Polanyi PhD. Drs. Stuart Strong and Gaza Jako worked with American Optical Laboratories to manufacture a Carbon Dioxide laser with an arm attachment. Excited by electricity, the laser beam produced by the excitement of the carbon dioxide gas molecules, traveled through an articulated arm and produced heat for tissue interaction. In 1971, Dr. R.R. Hall defined the tissue effects of the Carbon Dioxide laser, developing the theory of cell vaporization by the laser beam. In 1971, Dr. F. L'Esperance reported the use of the Nd: YAG laser on seven patients with various ophthalmological problems.

In 1972, Dr. G.J. Jako, M.D. used the Carbon Dioxide laser to remove benign lesions from vocal cords in humans. In 1975, the neurosurgeons using the CO/2 lasers to vaporize large tumors with little or no manipulation of the tumor. In 1977, Dr. J. Bellina adapted the CO/2 laser for use in Gynecology. In 1977, Johnson, et all, brought the use of the Nd: YAG laser to medicine. That same year several German physicians began using this application in Urology and Gastroenterology. In 1983, this laser was used to successfully ablate an esophageal cancer. The Nd: YAG modality was introduced in a pulsed mode in 1977 almost simultaneously, by Frankhauser in Switzerland, and Aron-Rosa in France, but not in the United States until 1980. In 1976, Dr. Thomas Dougherty, PhD. at Roswell Park in Buffalo, New York began working, using laser irradiation with an injectable dye, a photochemical reaction, as adjunctive therapy used in cancer treatment. The growth of lasers in medicine has barely touched the tip of the "iceberg." The future of lasers in medicine and surgery is expanding rapidly, and has implications on our practice as health care givers.

In 1985, Dr. Stephen N. Joffe and others, particularly in Japan, developed a Contact Laser used with sapphire quartz probes that began to revolutionize the use of the Nd: YAG laser.

In 1979, the International Laser Society was founded in Israel, and in 1980, the American Society for Laser Medicine and Surgery was founded. Many countries have established laser societies and come together at these meetings to share information, since that time lasers have proliferated in surgical and many medical disciplines.

Part 1
Technical Aspects of Lasers

CHAPTER 1
BASIC LASER BIOPHYSICS

Laser is an acronym that describes a process by which electrical energy is converted to light energy. It represents:

L ight
A mplification by the
S timulated
E mission of
R adiation

How does the laser work and why is its becoming one of the advanced technologies used in surgery and medicine today? A basic review of physics as applied to lasers will help in understanding the phenomena involved in laser technology.

Light is a form of electro-magnetic energy. The exact nature of light isn't understood, but has discrete characteristics of photon and waves. Primarily we look at light in the terms of wave characteristics. Those are:

Wavelength
Frequency
Velocity
Amplitude

Color is related to wavelength and changes in energy status. Some colors are detectable and others are invisible. Other wavelengths exit such as infrared and ultraviolet. Each wavelength has a particular property and each photon has a predictable color.

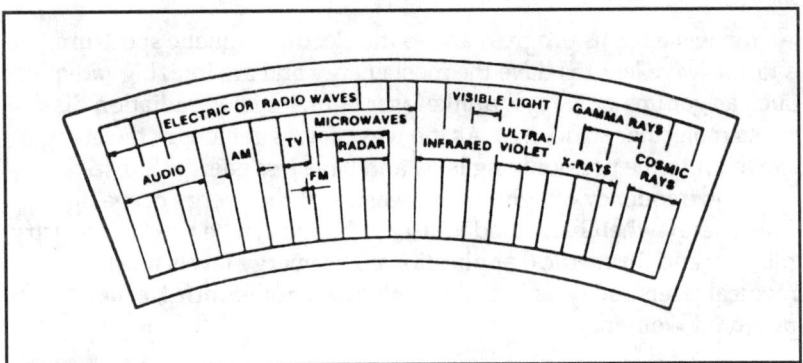

Figure 1.1
The Electro-Magnetic Spectrum

A **wavelength** is the distance between two successive crests and this determines the color. The wavelength of laser light is discussed at the nanometers level. A nanometer is 10^{-9} m and visible light waves are between 385 to 760 nanometers, crossing all the primary colors from **violet** to **red**.

The **frequency** of a wave is the number of waves passing a given point per second and is expressed in **cycles** or **hertz**. The shorter the wavelength the higher the frequency.

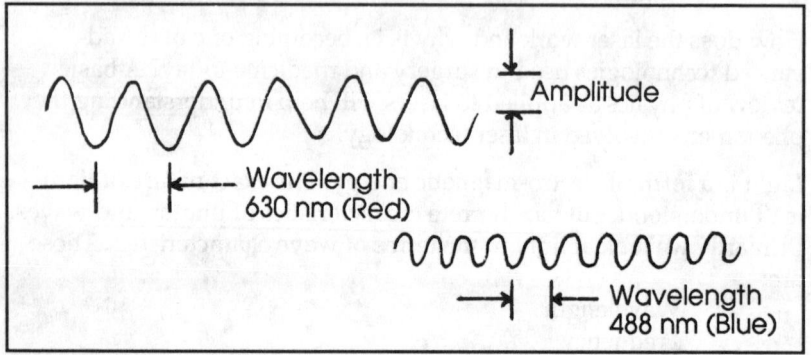

Figure 1.2
Wave Forms

The length and frequency are inversely related; as the wavelength increases or decreases, frequency decreases or increases, respectively. However, one can change the color of the light by changing the energy level of the photon.

As the wave forms progress across the electro-magnetic spectrum, the shorter wave lengths have the most energy and are ionizing radiation; such as gamma or X-rays, unlike laser light, ionizing radiation disrupts molecular structures. As the wave forms get longer the energy moved into the non-ionizing level and have less energy. Subsequently, frequency of light is the measure of the energy of the light. This energy when harnessed is laser light and can be used in industry, military and for medical applications. The energy levels used in medical lasers today, is non-absorptive and **not harmful, especially to pregnant women.**

Laser light differs from other light. To understand this phenomena the rules of **Quantum Mechanics** are reviewed. In an atom, the relationship between the electrons and the nucleus is described in terms of

Basic Laser Biophysics

energy levels. Quantum Mechanics predicts that these energy levels are discrete. Electrons normally occupy the lowest available energy levels. If two stimulated atoms collide, each will release its quantity of energy stimultaneously and in equal amounts. Electrons will stay in this higher energy level, or "excited-state," for a short time before dropping back to the original ground state or resting state.

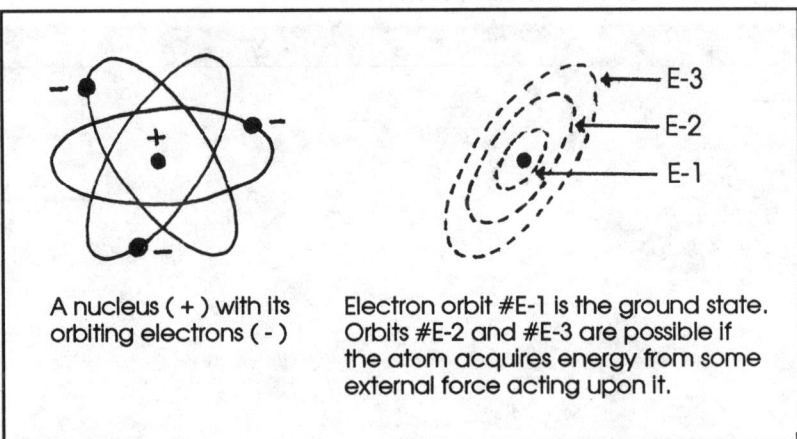

A nucleus (+) with its orbiting electrons (-)

Electron orbit #E-1 is the ground state. Orbits #E-2 and #E-3 are possible if the atom acquires energy from some external force acting upon it.

Figure 1.3
Stimulated Energy Levels

When these electrons drop to their original ground state, the process causes a **photon of light energy** to be **spontaneously emitted.**

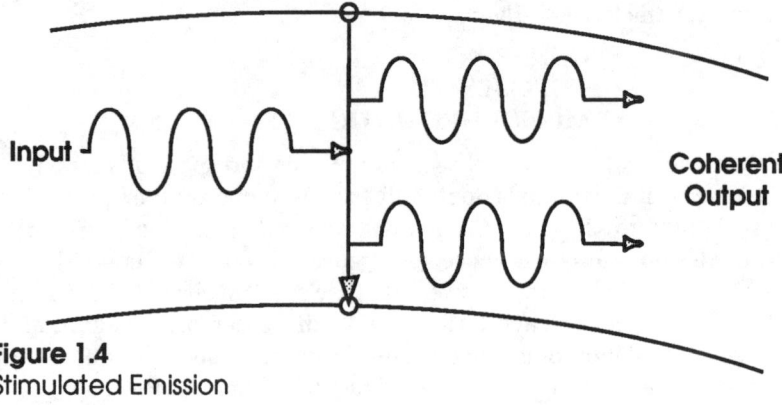

Figure 1.4
Stimulated Emission

An atom can be excited to a higher energy level by absorbing a photon, but only if the energy of the photon is equal to the energy difference between orbits. Excitement won't happen if the photon doesn't have the same energy, frequency, wavelength, and color. An electron in an excited state can be **stimulated** by another photon of precisely the correct energy, to undergo orbital decay and emit another **identical** photon. *A photon is a unit of light energy.* The result is two photons of equal wavelength leaving the atom together is exactly the same direction and perfectly in phase with each other begin **stimulated emission.** (see figure 1.4)

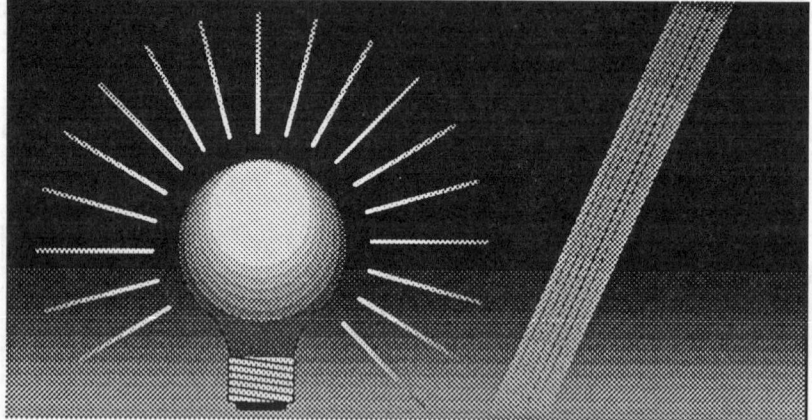

Figure 1.5
White Light vs Laser Light

Unlike, ordinary white light that is incoherent, with multiple divergent angles so it appears as white light and has difficulty being optically collimated (see figure 1.5) **stimulated emission** has three unique characteristics, they are:

- COHERENT
- COLLIMATED
- MONOCHROMATIC

When two photons are in phase, both in time and space, it's called *Coherence*. If the photons do not diverge from one another as they travel outward, they stay *Collimated*. The path of photons are parallel so there's no beam divergence. (see figure 1.5) When the emitted photons are of identical wavelength, they're *Monochromatic*. As the photons bounce back and forth, they'll strike other excited atoms and cause a population build-up or **"population inversion"** of photons all the same wavelength. For tissue interaction a minimum of one photon must be absorbed.

How does a laser work? There are four basic components of a laser:

- **Active Medium**
- **Excitation Mechanism**
- **Feedback Mechanism**
- **Output Couple**

Basic Laser Biophysics

Lasers are named by their **active medium**. The four types of lasers are:
- **Solid**
- **Gas**
- **Liquid**
- **Electronic**

Solid - State lasers use a lasing material distributed in a solid matrix. The ruby laser, using a ruby crystal, is in the visible red spectrum at 694 nanometers. This laser isn't efficient and is difficult to maintain. The Neodymium Yttrium Aluminum Garnet (abbreviated Nd: YAG) laser is invisible in the near infrared at 1060 nanometers. Other solid state lasers are in being developed using a variety of elements. These lasers require an optical power source such as flash lamps to excite the laser medium.

Gas lasers use a mixture of gases contained in a tube. **Argon** and **Krypton** gas lasers have multiple frequency emissions in the visible spectrum. The Argon laser is an ion gas, visible, green or green-blue, at 458-515 nanometers. Because of the wavelength property of the Argon beam, it can be used with fiberoptics. Krypton wavelength is strongest at 647 nanometers, red, but can also provide visible light through the yellow, orange spectrum. The **Helium-Neon** laser is visible and red at 632.8 nanometers. This laser wavelength is used as the co-axial or "aiming beam" for lasers in the infrared portion of the spectrum. The **Carbon Dioxide (CO_2)** laser uses molecular gas, is invisible, in the far infra red at 10,600 nanometers. CO_2 lasers are stable at low powers and currently the most efficient laser.

Liquid lasers use complex organic dye in a solution or suspension. The laser's feature is its **"tunibility."** The choice of dye and its concentration allows the production of laser light over a broad range of wavelengths.

Electronic lasers, called **diodes,** have two layers of semiconductor material **"sandwiched"** together emitting an intense beam of infrared light when energized by direct current. (This type is used in compact discs) These lasers are very small and have low power output at approximately 4-70 watts.

There are different modes of operation or **"excitation mechanisms"** that create energy in the active medium. The modes of operation is distinguished by the rate at which the energy is delivered.

- **Continuous wave** is a continuously radiating laser beam. The power density is constant with time.
- **Long-pulsed or pulsed lasers** operate in normal

pulse mode and have pulse durations of a few hundred micro-seconds to a few hundred milli-seconds. Femto seconds are 10^{-15} seconds, pico-seconds are 10^{-12} seconds and nano-seconds are 10^{-9} seconds.

- **Rapid pulse lasers** operate similarly to the pulsed mode, but are capable to pulse rates that range from 10 to 1,000 pulses per second.
- **Mode-locked lasers** affect the characteristics of the output beam. When the phases of different frequency modesare synchronized (locked together) the modes will interfere with one another to give a "beat" effect. This will result in laser output as regularly spaced pulsations, each having a duration of pico-seconds to nano-seconds. A mode-locked laser can deliver extremely high peak powers.
- **Q-switched lasers** store energy until the population inversion reaches a certain level. These use a shutter technique to prevent laser emission until the desired time, then the energy is released very quick into one "giant" pulse. The "Q" represents the quality factor of the laser cavity.
- **Frequency doubling** is transforming light of one wavelength to light of another wavelength. By passing the beam of one wavelength through a non-linear crystal, a new wavelength is generated called a "harmonic" (like changing to different keys when playing a musical instrument). We can take Nd: YAG at 1060 nm, pass it through a non-linear medium as Alexandrite or a Potassium-Teonyl-Phosphate crystal (KTP) creating a new wavelength. The second harmonic green light at 532 nm or called "frequency doubling" (taking the frequency of the wave form and dividing it in half) by creating this wave form you've greater divergence of your beam "spot size" and reduce power output. Other harmonics, third, ourth, could also be generated.

Each medium has different **excitation mechanisms.** A pumping system gives energy to the atoms of the lasing medium, exciting them to give up photons. An optical pump uses photons supplied by another source such as continuous glow lamps or flash lamps to transfer energy to the lasing medium. Direct current from 200 to

Basic Laser Biophysics

25,000 volts excites lasers electrically. Also, radio frequency can be used, this may interfere with monitors and other electrical equipment in the operating room, however, most lasers have protective baffling to prevent micro-electrical energy leakage.

The **feedback mechanism** is the key to the amplification of light produced by stimulated emission. The optical cavity or resonating chamber has reflective mirrors at both ends; one is partially reflective. Light is amplified as its moves through the active medium. A small fraction of light is emitted spontaneously along the axis of the cavity in a direction so it reflects back and forth between the mirrors and passes through the active medium repeatedly. The light is in phase with itself after one round trip between the mirrors. The resonating chamber accumulates the intensity of the photons until the waves reach a threshold " gain " and finally exit one end of the chamber.

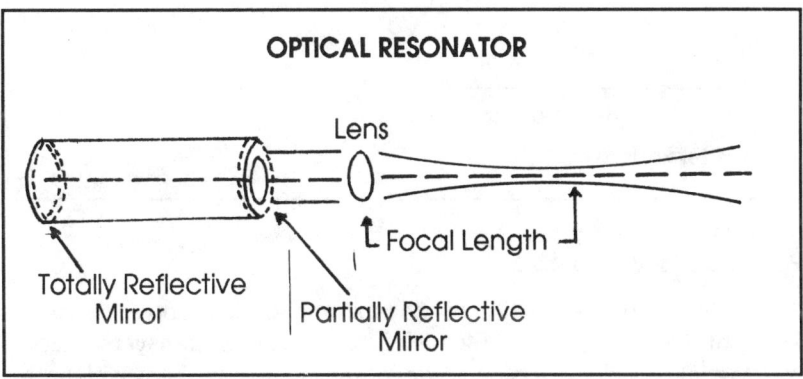

Figure 1.6
Resonating Chambers with Output Coupler

The special mirrors are the **output coupler** and are used at the each end of the resonating chamber. Once excitation of the photons has begun in the chamber, a shutter mechanism is activated and light waves must be released to be functional. As the amplification process continues, a part of the waves (radiation) will escape through the partially reflecting mirror. The mirrors in the optical cavity must be precisely aligned for the light beams to parallel the axis. A narrow concentrated beam of pure coherent light is formed, the laser beam.

Power density is the single, essential factor in effective operation of lasers. The term **power (P)** is related to watts or heat output produced by the laser system. **Energy (E)** is a product of power (watts) and its duration (seconds) on tissue to have effective vaporization or coagulation. Tissue injury is directly related to time and power, and not directly related to energy. The powers density formula is, **watts/cm$_2$**. <u>The surface area of the spot size and the power</u> **(watts)** determines the **power density.** (see figure 1.7)

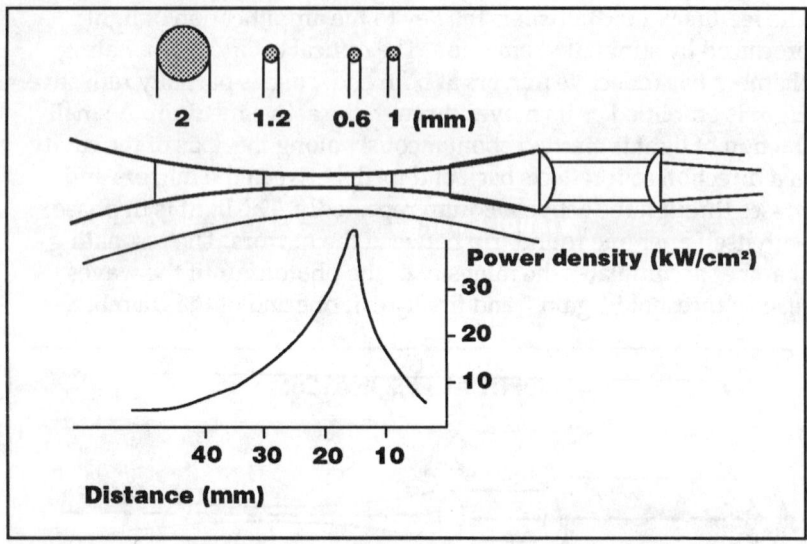

Figure 1.7
Power Density/Spot Size

Power density is the function of spot size and applied power in watts. The spot size is determined by the length of the lens, transverse electro-magnetic mode (gaussian curve) of the beam, and the wavelength of the laser. This power density is called **"fluence"** and is a <u>measure of total energy</u> directed to the tissue during treatment. This energy delivered to the target tissue has direct correlation with the thermal effect on tissue, and determines whether the laser will coagulate, vaporize or cut the target. (see figure 1.8)

Lenses are interchangable and the spot size can be controlled to affect the wavelengths. Spot size partically determines the thermal effect and can be controlled through special optics to do precise medica procedures. Mode refers to the distribution of power over the spot area and determines the preciseness of the spot size. The fundamental TEM oo shows even power distribution over the spot. (refer to figure 1.7)

Basic Laser Biophysics

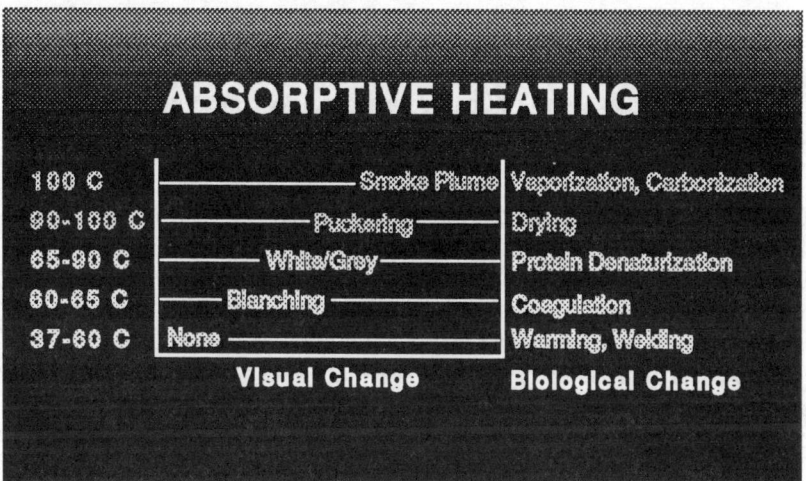

Figure 1.8
Absorption Correlations

The **transverse electro-magnetic mode** refers to the distribution of energy across the wave form of the laser beam. The energy is most intense in the beam center and decreases in intensity across a laser beam profile. It's necessary to understand variations in the energy distribution for optimum use of power density for tissue destruction. The concept restricts damage to healthy tissues in the area of impact by limiting the time exposure of the beam.

Power density can be calculated and a chart of each physicians preference kept on file. When the beam is used as a cutting tool, high power density with a small spot size will incise tissue and avoid thermal effect on surrounding healthy tissue. When coagulation is desired, defocusing of the laser beam increases the spot size for larger area of thermal impact and vaporization.

SUMMARY

Lasers are complex, with optical resonators, incorporating various lasing mediums, mirrors, lens, and have stimulated energy and cooling mechanisms to produce intense beams of energy.

LASER is an acronym describing a process that converts matter into light energy. Its stands for **Light Amplification by the Stimulated Emission of Radiation**. The theory was first described by Einstein in the early 1900's, but it wasn't until 1958 that amplification by stimulated emission was described by Schawlow and Townes, using microwaves. In 1960 Dr. Theodore Maiman, also a physicist, used a ruby crystal to build a laser, and in 1962 this laser was used in medicine.

Lasers use light in a controlled form of electro-magnetic energy, having such light characteristics as wavelengths, frequency, velocity, and amplitude. Laser light differs from white light, using high energy levels that stimulate the emission of photons in a straight line (collimated), in phase (coherent), and monochromatic (same wavelength).

The laser has four basic components; and active medium, an excitation mechanism, a feedback mechanism, and an output coupler. The laser works as the active medium is excited, and the photons bounce back and forth between two mirrors increasing photon population. A stream of photons escapes through the partially reflecting mirror supplying light of one color, straight beam, and in phase. The power density ($P = watts/cm_2$) of the laser beam is the single, essential factor in the effective operation of lasers. The transverse electro-magnetic mode (TEM_{oo}) shows the distribution of power of the spot size. High power density is used for small spot size in the cutting mode; to coagulate or vaporize you defocus the beam and reduce the power output. Put this together in one highly technical instrument makes the use of laser in surgery an invaluable tool.

CHAPTER 2
TYPES OF LASERS

There are primarily three types of lasers used biomedically:

1. Argon / Krypton
2. Carbon Dioxide (CO2)
3. Neodymium Yittrium Aluminum Garnet (Nd: YAG)

Other lasers that have been used in medicine and surgery, but to a lesser degree, are:

1. Ruby
2. Tunable Dye
3. Flash Pumped Dye
4. Helium Neon
5. Semi - Conductor
6. Excimer

Lasers that may introduced in medicine soon are; **Erbrium YAG, Hydrogen Fluoride, Nd: YLF, TEA CO2 and the Free Electron.** Lasers are known by the material used as their **active medium** and are named by wavelength and power output. For proper choice of lasers, several, important parameters must be considered, such as; wavelength, power and energy characteristics, and coefficient of absorption. These characteristics are important for determining tissue vaporization or coagulation. Each type of laser will be discussed considering the active medium for lasing.

GAS LASERS

ARGON-ION lasers produce the highest visible power levels. The most prominent Argon wavelengths are the 488 and 514.5 nm levels. These wavelengths are easily transmitted through clear, aqueous tissue or material. Also, certain pigmented tissue such as melanin and hemoglobin will absorb Argon laser light, effectively.
To dissipate the large amount of heat generated, Argon-ion laser tubes are water or air cooled. The water must flow at a certain pressure and sufficient rate, otherwise bailing happens along the tube. The bailing effects make cavity vibrations and in turn will make amplitude and frequency instabilities.

Pulsed and continuous wave versions of Argon-ion lasers are available. The average power output typically available is between 4-20 watts. The Argon laser beam can be transmitted through optical fibers.

CARBON DIOXIDE lasers offers a range from low to high power and has high efficiency in the far infrared wavelength for use in the medical applications of laser therapy. Carbon Dioxide lasers are the most efficient lasers and can produce power outputs of 1-100 watts and emit invisible light in the infrared region of 10,600 nanometers. The principal difference between the CO_2 laser and the other gas lasers is that the optics must be coated or made of special material being reflective or transmissive at the far infrared wavelength.

The **optical resonator** has a pair of long radius curvature mirrors, with multi-laser dielectric reflective coating. Additives to the CO_2 gas increase the operating efficiency, the most common composition being a mixture of helium, nitrogen, and carbon dioxide. The CO_2 laser beam can't, at present, be transmitted through fiberoptics, although CO_2 fibers are in the developmental stage. CO_2 lasers are coupled with an operating microscope and rigid endoscopes for use as a precision instrument, and the depth of tissue damage can be controlled. The CO_2 laser is well established as a surgical tool for incision, vaporizing and coagulation of tissue for many surgical procedures. Focused to a fine point, it can incise tissue. Defocused, as the energy is spread over a wider area, it can coagulate or vaporize tissue. New technology has been recently introduced using **"sealed tube"** technology. The CO_2 gas mixture is sealed in a laser tube with a catalyst to rebind the CO_2 molecule. This laser. Needs no external laser gas supply.

SOLID STATE LASERS

NEODYMIUM YITTRIUM ALUMINUM GARNET (Nd: YAG) laser, also called YAG, is a solid state laser whose active medium is a crystal doped with an impurity ion, a substance similarly used to create synthetic diamonds. The solid crystal is optically pumped by flash lamps placed directly next to the laser rod. The solid crystal is stimulated to emit laser light in the near infrared region of 1064 nm. The YAG laser can produce power output form 0 to 150 watts, transmitted through a fiberoptic system. The laser must be cooled by air or circulating water pressure, as high power operation caused thermal expansion of the crystal that may change the mode.

The YAG laser beam can be transmitted through a clear liquid medium that allows its being used in fluid filled cavities or clear solid materials. The YAG laser light isn't color dependent so it may be absorbed by almost any tissue that's unclear. The physical characteristics of the YAG laser beam are; it has a high degree of scattering in the tissue, and thermal coagulation and necrosis may extend beyond the impact site to about 4 mm, so precise control may not be possible.

Types of Lasers

These characteristics make the Nd: YAG laser an excellent tool for coagulation and ablation. Since the arrival of contact laser surgery with the use of synthetic sapphire probes or scalpels used with the YAG laser has returned precision of cutting to this modality, with less thermal necrosis.

The **Ruby laser** is also a solid state laser in the visible range of 694 nanometers. This laser system was used early in Ophthalmology and is still being used occasionally in Dermatology. This laser has the capability of generating large fields of energy on impact, making a shock wave effect. This high energy can cause increase tissue damage, has power output between 10 and 100 milli-joules, and is used in a pulsed mode. This laser system is difficult to maintain and isn't being used routinely in the medical field.

LIQUID OR DYE LASERS

LIQUID LASERS have unique advantages for certain applications and provide a narrow band of highly coherent light that has a wide range of uses, including spectroscopy, cell sorting, and counting devices used in the laboratory. Using the dye laser, the output is tunable over a significant frequency range. The active medium has organic dyes dissolved in a solvent, usually ethyl alcohol. When the dye is excited by external sources of short wavelength, such as the Argon laser, it stimulates the dye and causes it to lase in different wavelengths.

When used to treat patients, the liquid or dye lasers are used with photo-active drugs given to the patient before laser treatment. The laser beam is coupled with fiberoptics and by using varying types of dye with the tuning system, different wavelengths can be obtained. When using the particular photosensitizer, such as a hematoporphyrin derivative, the tunable dye laser is used at 633 nanometers. When the patient has been premedicated with the photosensitizer and exposed to a specific wavelength, an oxidative process happens.

This process produces a photochemical reaction cellular deactivation and tissue death. Dye lasers can be pulsed across several wavelengths and are being used in several specialties such as; Ophthalmology, for macular degenerative diseases, Dermatology, superficial and deep vascular lesions, Urology and General Surgery, to fragment a variety of calculi, depending on the structure of the stone.

ELECTRONIC LASERS

RADIO FREQUENCY is used to excite the active medium which is usually CO_2 in a sealed laser tube. The wavelength is in the 10,600 nm range with a power output of 0 to 20 watts. These lasers are usually air cooled and don't need an external gas supply.

SEMI-CONDUCTOR is a type of solid state laser commercially available. Its is very efficient and very small, well suited for the industrial application of lasers. These lasers are currently being used as light sources for fiberoptic communication. These lasers will be used in combination with computers to enhance our ability to introduce valuable diagnostic tools.

OTHER LASERS

New lasers that may be introduced into medicine and surgery are:

1. EXICIMER
This pulsed laser emits a wavelength of between 193/ 248 and 351 nm, depending on the lasermedium. The laser medium. The laser medium used for the Excimer laser are excited dimers of noble gases such as, Argon Fluoride or Xenon Fluoride gas. Photon energy is con verted to electrical excitation, leading to the breaking of the molecular bonds of the cellular structure without the energy degrading into heat. This laser beam can be delivered through optic fibers.

2. ERIBRIUM YAG
Has a wavelength of 1094 nm and may be more effective for some tissue interaction. The absorption wavelength of water is 1090 nm.

SHORT PULSE LASERS

1. TRANSVERSE EXCITED ATMOSPHERE $C0_2$
Short pulse ablation causes minimal tissue damage andthe physicians will have greater control.

2. FREQUENCY DOUBLED YAG LASERS
Using a KTP crystal (Potassium Teonyl Phosphate) producing visible light at 532 nm that can be delivered through a 600 micron quartz fiber. This produces a beam of lime green light with 0.3 to 2 mm depth of penetra tion, absorbed in reddish pigments. The output energy is limited to 10 - 12 watts.

3. FREE ELECTRON
Lasers are reaching into the future. The Strategic Defense Initiative Program has allocated about 60 million dollars for research in the field. Early experiment showed the electron beam from a linear accelerator running through a magnetic field could produce a narrow emission of spontaneous radiation. Can this be applied to medicine? Only the future will tell us.

SUMMARY

The use of lasers in medicine and surgery is new and evolutionary and there will be 298 million dollars spent in laser sales by 1990. The laser adds a versatile and viable tool to the physician's armamentarium for increased quality of care and other choices for treatment of various disease entities.

Surgical application using the primary lasers available in medicine today are broad and varying, applicable in most disciplines. The CO_2 laser is now a well accepted surgical tool for vaporizing and incising tissue. The CO_2 laser is being used in Neurosurgery, Gynecology, Otolaryngology, General Surgery, Dermato-Plastic Surgery, Podiatry and limited use in other specialties such as; Orthopedics, Urology, and Thoracic Surgery.

The **Argon** laser is used in Ophthalmology, Gastroenterology, and Dermatology for its ability to do eye procedures inside and intact globe and for its selective absorption by pigmented tissue.

The **Nd: YAG** laser's primary use is for its coagulation properties and ability being used through a liquid medium or clear material. It's increased use in Genitourinary, Gastroenterology, Pulmonary, General Surgery, Ophthalmology, and Gynecology.

New lasers are being introduced everyday and will accepted across all specialties giving the physician optimal wave lengths for selective absorption in tissue to minimize his treatment modality.

This list is limited however, as laser technology becomes acceptable in the medical and surgical applications as a primary instrument for treatment. The use is only limited by the mind of the user.

CHAPTER 3

TISSUE EFFECTS OF LASERS

Once the pathophysiological considerations of the etiology have been determined, the type of therapy needed for that specific indication may be better treated with the laser.

The most commonly used lasers in medicine and surgery are:

- Argon-ion   488-515 nm
- Carbon Dioxide   10,600 nm
- Nd: YAG   1,064 nm

Each type of laser has a different biological effect on tissue, so each has varying applications. Lasers are a special form of light and obey all the physics and photochemical laws of light.

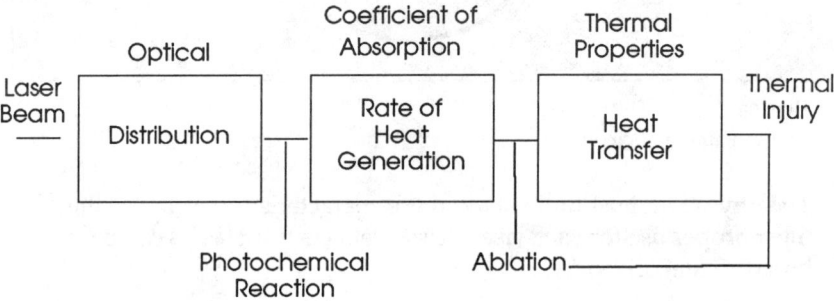

Figure 3.1
Steps of Laser Tissue Interaction

Grotthus - Draper's law states" *that light must be absorbed to provide energy for photochemical or photobiological reaction or nothing will happen* " (see figure 3.1) As laser light interacts with tissue it's either absorbed, reflected, transmitted or scattered. If the light will affect the tissue it must be absorbed. When it's reflected or transmitted through tissue, it's little effect until it reaches the target. When scattered over a broad area its effect will be diffused. (see figure 3.2, p. 20)

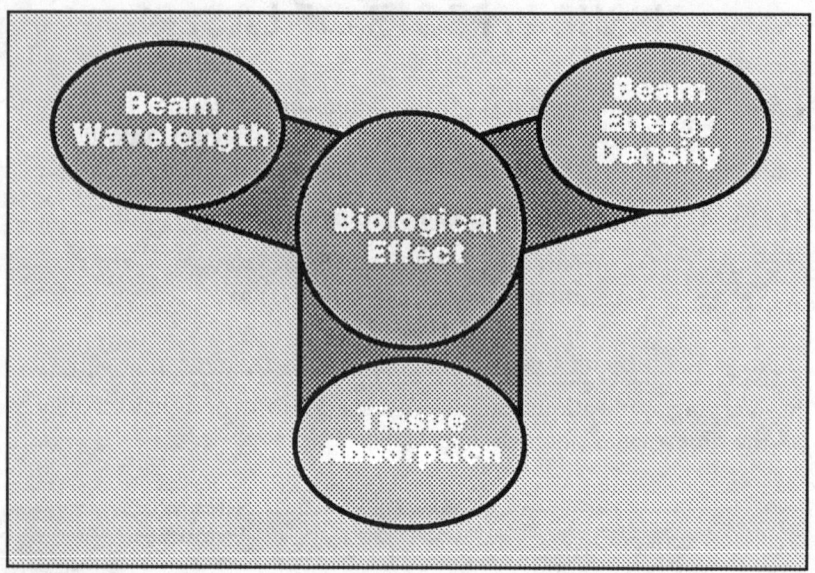

Figure 3.2
Tissue Interaction

The physician must understand these characteristics to choose the most proper use for each laser. Tissue effects from lasers can be broadly categorized:

>   **Vaporization**
>   **Cutting**
>   **Ablation**
>   **Coagulation**
>   **Hemostasis**
>   **Necrosis**

For cutting, the laser beam is focused to a fine spot for preciseness and localization of tissue damage. The laser is vaporizing the tissue. The cellular water is heated beyond the boiling point, causing destruction of the cellular protein with pressure build up within the cell. The rise of intra-cellular temperature and pressure makes the cell to explode, giving off steam and debris. (refer to figure 3.3) The explosion of the cellular content is seen as a **"laser plume" (smoke).** However, tissue damage is very limited.

Tissue Effects of Lasers

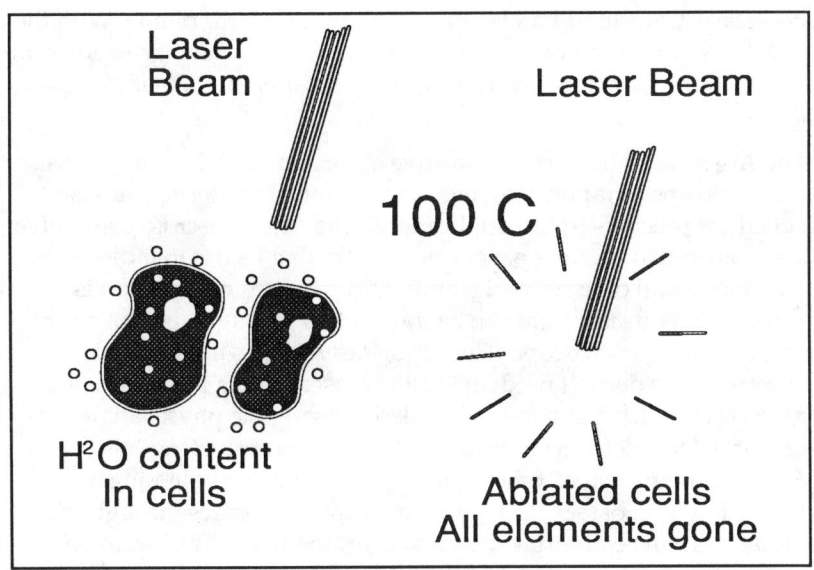

Figure 3.3
Photoablation of a Cell

As the laser beam cuts through tissue it seals small vessels and the lymphatics, creating a dry surgical field. The sealing effect on the tissue usually reduces edema, scarring and stenosis. The depth of the cut is determined by the power density and the time the beam is applied to the tissue. Some laser beams penetrate the tissue and cellular membrane and continues to travel into the tissue behind it. A backstop must be used to prevent damage to next tissue. With the CO_2 laser, the backstop is usually wet sponges. Cottonoids, fluid, quartz or titanium rods.

The technique for vaporization of tissue is to use a defocused spot size with high power density. The advantage of vaporization is in precisely removing larges masses of tissue one layer at a time from delicate structures such as blood vessels and nerves. Laser vaporization only happens in a dry field as the energy will boil the blood and no tissue effect will happen. The laser produces cellular debris and smoke when used in a defocused mode and a smoke evacuation (suction) system must be used to clear the surgical field. Laser plume is noxious and may contain mutagenic cellular debris. The plume must be evacuated however, not directly in the central vacuum system. Use either an evacuation system designed for this purpose or a plume filter connected directly to the central vacuum system, is necessary. Canister filters aren't enough to filter laser plume. With the CO_2 laser, you're lasing what you see with limited damage to adjacent tissue. The Argon and Nd: YAG laser have different scientific applications.

The **Argon** laser has a color sensitive absorption rate in living tissue. It's limited penetration combined with minimal scattering, and isn't suited for precise surgical applications. The Argon laser is coagulative and has limited thermal penetration, restricting its use to indications where removal of tissue and simultaneous limited coagulation is wanted. Argon laser light can be transmitted through fiberoptics or and operating microscope. The Argon laser light is in the visible spectrum and doesn't need an ancillary laser aiming beam. Krypton gas is being added to many Argon laser, giving the physician the use of a broader spectrum of wavelengths. **Krypton** wavelength is 554 to 647 nm moving across yellow, orange to red visible light ranges in tissue. Krypton passes through clear media and passes through red tissue and can be absorbed by darker caraton tissue. It's less intense, making slower coagulation of blood and tissue. This laser is often used in the macular area of the retina.

The laser best suited for coagulation is the **Nd: YAG** laser. With the Nd: YAG laser, there's thermal penetration and low absorption in tissue, making it suitable as a coagulator. The Nd: YAG laser light can be transmitted through fiberoptics and used with endoscopes, handpieces, or the operating microscope. Time is a factor when manipulating tissue effects with the YAG laser, usually in the non-contact mode. The introduction of synthetic sapphire quartz probes or scalpels used with the Nd: YAG laser change the principle use of this laser. Using low power settings the contact probes provide the capability of cutting, coagulating, vaporization, and interstitial irradiation with the contact YAG laser. This development allows controlled manipulation of the laser beam and restores the tactile feedback to the surgeon. The beam can be used in a "pulsed" or "continuous" mode. The Nd: YAG and CO_2 lasers' beams are in the invisible spectrum and an aiming laser beam, usually helium neon (HeNe), is used for controlled alignment of the laser beam.

The steam and cellular debris that stay in the path of the laser beam are the by products of vaporization, called a plume. Laser energy causes rapid temperature elevation of intra-cellular water, resulting in cell wall explosion. Although, there have been studies done to analyze the plume content for intact DNA of viral particals and carcinogenics,

Tissue Effects of Lasers

no conclusive proof has been proven to show the viability of the particals at high or low powers or particular laser wavelengths. The contact YAG laser surgery causes less thermal necrosis in tissue and doesn't cause tissue necrosis for more than 0.5 mm depth of penetration. The effects of lasers on tissue aren't totally conclusive and research is continuing.

Currently, the principal known effects on tissue are:

- Vaporization
- Coagulation
- Absence of fibrosis and stenosis
- Sterilization of tissue at the operative site
- Seals lymphatics, reducing dissemination of malignant cells
- Little damage to adjacent tissue, reducing edema
- Color selective
- Selective photochemical response
- Apparent reduced post-operative pain
- Reduced blood loss

SUMMARY

The laser chosen for use by the physician has varying applications and each will have a different biological effect on tissue. The advantages of laser use are categorized in broad terms, they're; vaporization, coagulation, or ablation. The skilled surgeon will know how to used each modality appropriately for his/her surgical discipline and may use one or all during a procedure. However, the advantages may have more applicability for quality patient care.

CHAPTER 4

LASER SAFETY

Lasers have been used in medicine and surgery worldwide. A laser can concentrate a high energy output into a small, collimated beam, this could potentially be dangerous. The future of laser therapy lies with the user, and it is imperative that for the safety of patients, physician and other medical personnel, all understand each laser wavelength according to its safe use in medical applications. Manufacturers of lasers are also responsible for the safety of medical lasers. Lasers are non-ionizing (non-absorptive and aren't dangerous to pregnant women), and produce beams of light energy that can be divided into two broad hazard categories. Those in the optical range of 400-1400 nm, where a refocused image to the retina may cause damage. The other is the ultraviolet and infrared, and invisible light sources.

Lasers are a medical device and fall under the jurisdiction of the Medical Device Regulations as published in the Federal Register, Volume 40, Part II, July 30, 1975. Other sources for laser safety guidelines are: American National Standards Institute Z136.1 and the newly released Z136.3. "Guidelines for Safe Laser Use in Medical Facilities," U. S. Department of Health and Human Services, 21 CFR, Part 58 and Public Health Service manual Chapter 1-14 and the National Institute of Health Manual Issuance 4206 and 6000-3-4.58. There are several government regulatory groups whoare involved in laser safety, they are:

- Food and Drug Administration
- American National Standards Institute
- Occupational Safety and Health Administration
- Bureau of Radiological Health
- International Electro-technical Commission
- American Conferences of Governmental Industrial Hygienists

In 1976, the F.D.A. issued a mandate defining medical devices and the process for their development. The law has classified medical products into three groups according to how difficult it is to assure safety. These classifications are:

- Class I   Subject to general controls
- Class II All devices for which general controls arenot enough
- Class III Consists of implants and life support ing devices

Class II devices must be approved for safety and effectiveness before they can be marketed. Lasers are Class III medical devices and have been divided into four sub-classifications:

- Class 1   Lasers are enclosed systems and don't emit hazardous levels.
- Class 2   Lasers are limited to visible light and are safe for momentary viewing.
- Class 3   Lasers that call for procedural controls and protective equipment.
- Class 4   Lasers are potentially hazardous, could produce fire, skin burns, or are capable of diffuse reflections, with probability of retinal exposure.

Being able to use lasers in medicine and surgery they must be approved by the F.D.A. (Section 520g) that showed significant studies were undertaken to develop the effectiveness and safety to use on human subjects. Being allowed to complete research on humans subjects application must be made to the F.D.A.

Information needed to be submitted; detailed criteria and supporting hypothesis regarding the study, who's sponsoring the study (physician group or agency); definition of the significant risks; explanation of expected outcomes, the responsible party, who's on the institutional review board, method of monitoring the study, and maintenance of records. When this information has been reviewed by the F.D.A. and the project approved for investigation, an IDE (**Investigational Device Exempt**) number is assigned to the project. When all the data is submitted, reviewed, can be replicated and shown being efficacious with little or no risk to human subjects a **PMA (Pre Market Approval)** document is issued. The public, other manufacturers or investigators can challenge, comment or request a hearing within 30 days. If nothing happens, approval for the medical device or procedure is

Laser Safety

done and the F.D.A. has the authority to review, inspect or investigate the researchers facility or records whenever, without prior notification. Another way to receive approval for the new medical devices, i.e., lasers, is to file a **510K document** that submits substantive data that the instrument or procedures are as good as or better that what exists in the market place. With these controls and bureaucratic agencies as "watch dogs," we as prudent health care providers must establish criteria for approval and compliance in our facilities.

Safety rules protect the patient and the user and are established by the Laser Committee. Established recommended criteria being considered are:

- Medical staff education and privilege approval criteria and process.
- Education of the nursing and support staff.
- Appointment of the Laser Safety Officer
- Approved Policies and Procedures.
- Job descriptions of laser operators.

The Joint Commission on the Accrediation for Hospitals 1986 guidelines, section on the "Governing Body," makes recommendations "for credentialing not only physicians, but individuals providing patient care services, to assure all patients are provided with quality care. JCAH further sates there should be methods implemented to monitor and evaluate this care."

Education criteria should be established by a medical staff committee, and the criteria defined should be realistic for physician compliance and monitored by the Laser Safety Officer. Until the graduating resident/nurse has finished the study of lasers, the biophysics, tissue pathophysiology, application in their particular specialty, and the safe use of the lasers in their practice, another mechanism, credentialing, certifies to his/her colleagues and the public a degree of recognized ability and knowledge.

Credentialing in the process to control access to difficult and complex intrumentation and techniques. Credentialing, belongs within the institution and should be delegated to a multi-disciplined committee. The composition of this committee should be those who will use laser techniques in their daily practice. The committee is usually formulated and directed by the facilities executive committee to develop written criteria and oversee approved regulations to ensure the safe use of the instrumentation and/or technique.

Learning, experiences for physicians are available through many established didactic and clinical courses through-out the United States. The recommended criteria could include:

1. Completion of an approved basic laser course that provides a stipulated number of hours for both didactic and "hands-on" clinical experience in animate objects, in a laboratory setting.

   a. a documented certificate awarded for successful completion of the course.

2. Participation in a limited preceptor or proctor program in the physician/nursing speciality under the direction of an experienced laser physician/nurse, either within or without of the hospital's setting.

   a. a letter or documentation form is submitted on the completion of the preceptor or proctor program.

3. Attendance at a formal in-service program conducted by the manufacturer on the operation and safety features of the laser and related equipment.

4. Repetition of the above sequence should new laser wavelengths be acquired.

5. Submit criteria for the quality assurance or peer review committee to randomly review laser utilization by accredited physicians within the facility.

Nursing certification should be established in the same prescribed manner, however, there should be several additions for nursing credentialing criteria, they are:

1. Develop standards for nursing practice during laser procedures.

2. Develop a patient education process.

3. Orientation process developed for nursing and other personnel, regarding laser safety.

4. Nursing documentation of laser therapy.

5. Develop a patient evaluation process.

6. Develop and establish discharge criteria.

Laser Safety

To reference the safety guidelines we look at the ANSI Z136.3, addendum for medical facility laser safety. The **Laser Safety Officer (LSO)** is appointed and approved by the medical executive committee. The LSO is responsible for establishing and monitoring laser safety for the institution. The LSO job description should include a general statement of responsibilities, environmental control criteria, and reporting mechanisms. The LSO must have the knowledge and understanding of the technical characteristics of all laser systems, assess potential laser hazards, understand medical applications to ensure laser safety in the clinical setting, report all incidents and plan for the prevention of recurring accidents. The LSO participates in the education and orientation of the physicians and nursing staff, and is a member of the facilities Safety Committee.

With a broad spectrum of potential hazards each health care facility must develop laser safety criteria that will be functional and accepted practice by physicians and user personnel. Laser safety criteria have been recommended by several governmental agencies and described by each speciality in their literature and easily adopted for hospital and physician office practice.

To manage laser safety and safe practice, the user should attend a laser safety and user training program. The training program should include:

- basic laser biophysics
- safety control measures
- medical indications and tissue effects
- applications of laser wavelengths for each specialty
- technical understanding of the used of each laser
- trouble shooting techniques
- documentation of laser use and maintenance
- patient and personnel education

As laser proliferate into all area of health care a body of experts, practitioners who uses lasers in their daily practice, to include administrative, nursing and engineering personnel, should be established. Medical staff by-laws may need to be reviewed to establish this group as a functional committee for quality assurance of the program. The **"Laser Committee"** has several functions:

1. Develop physician education criteria and participate inthe approval process.
2. Establish laser safety policies.
3. Approved laser usage procedures and the documentation process.

4. Help in the training of other physicians and laser support personnel.
   5. Develop the laser safety officer's job description and appoint the proper person to that position.
   6. Develop a quality assurance monitoring tool.

Laser safety is the responsibility of the health care institution and recommended guidelines covering all areas where lasers are used should be developed, as standard operating procedures.

Lasers used in the operating room are in a controlled environment and are being used by trained personnel. Understanding all the safety measures, having inter-locks on the doors limits access to the operating room. Current guidelines allow the LSO to make the final decision whether inter-locks will be installed. Signs posted on each entrance and personnel education should reduce the hazard of being exposed to laser light emission, unexpectedly.

However, when the laser is being used outside the controlled environment, i.e. ; endoscopy suites, physician's office or a clinic treatment area, safety latches or door inter-locks may be needed to prevent unexpected entry into the laser usage area. A controlled disconnect switch should be installed to deactivate the laser should emergency admission of personnel be needed.

The laser safety signs should be large and visibly placed at the entrance to the laser room. Also, all laser systems must be labeled by the American National Standard Institute guidelines.

Viewing windows should be covered or incorporated some means to attenuate laser radiation. Industrial grade laminated "day/dark" shades can be installed on the within the viewing window. (inside prevents any one from "peeking") The use of louvers inside a double window pane is recommended and cost justified only during a construction or renovation project.

Environmental hazards that may call for specific safety considerations resulting from specular reflection of the laser beam. The hazard of specular reflection is determined by diffuse laser wavelengths, optical surfaces, or because of light gathering capabilities of optical instrumentation, i.e., microscopes, or endoscopic instruments.

Surgical instruments used during laser procedures should have a dull finish, preferably anodized to reduce inadvertent or divergent reflections that may cause eye or skin injury.

Laser Safety

There are specific hazards in the use of lasers in the medical field. A description of these risks, in declining order, follows:

I. Burns

    A. Fire, either intra or extra luminal, elastomer endotracheal tubes, carrying gases that support combustion.

    B. Ignition of rectal gas expelled by the patient during surgery.

    C. Ignition of the endoscopic material in oxygen enriched atmosphere.

    D. Ignition or vaporization of surgical draping material.

    E. Combustion or ignition of solutions used in the surgical field.

II. Accidental trauma to unintended targets.

    A. Perforation of tissue other than the target tissue.

    B. Injury to nerves, brain, or spinal cord tissue.

    C. Injury to cornea, sclera, or retina.

    D. Injury from accidental thermal penetration.

III. Inappropriate or unskilled use.

    A. Use of laser on unknown histology.

    B. Excessive or delayed thermal necrosis form prolonged laser irradiation.

    C. Other injuries incurred by unskilled or untrained user.

    D. Equipment malfunction.

The administration of the facility where lasers are used must provide adequate supervision for development, implementation and maintenance of the laser safety policy and procedures. Administrative responsibility extends to the medical-legal implications of its utilization within the institution. Potential legal implications fall into several categories; they are; alleged negligence by the user, failure to get informed consent, and corporate negligence for inadequate supervision of the program.

The components of malpractice are; "duty" or "standard of care" owed by care providers, breech of duty or standard care, and resulting damages to the individual. These components need to be established by an expert witness during litigation. Another concern is the lack of concensus among experts in the laser field.

Liability can be minimized by the development and implementation of an approved laser safety protocol. Hospitals must establish educational criteria and uniformly enforce compliance to approved policies and procedures. A mechanism to regularly review laser utilization for quality assurance control.

There are several general rules for laser safety that should be followed:
1. Knowledge, of laser characteristics must be understood before operation of the equipment.
2. Never fire the laser until beam pathways have been established.
3. User education must happen before the use of therapeutic laser use on living tissue.
4. All laser policies and procedures developed and approved before utilization.
5. All inservices provided by the manufacturer finished.

Lasers are being installed in many clinical settings; Operating Rooms, Ambulatory Surgery Units, Endoscopy Suites, Clinics, and Physician's Offices. Quality patient care includes safety. Nurses must expand their knowledge to include all aspects of laser safety as these policies and procedures will apply to all area with little change. Persons chosen to work with laser systems should have mature judgement and reliability, receive laser education and training, understand the safety parameters and be aware of all laser hazards that may happen.

Persons near the laser and the emitted beams includes patients, staff and physicians. Proper protective equipment refers to eyewear, these are goggles or glasses of a specific optical density for each laser use. All protected eye wear must have the optical density labeled for use with each laser by the Bureau of Radiation Health, requirements.

Laser Safety 33

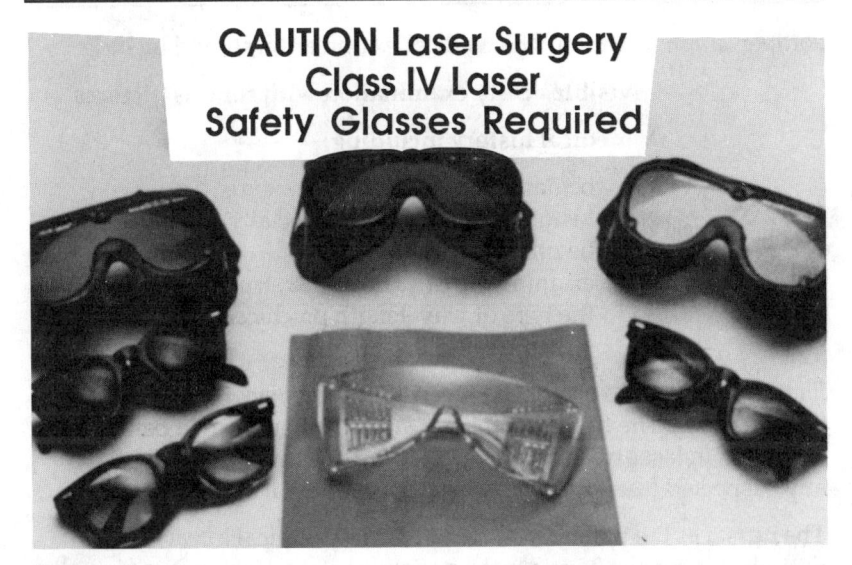

**CAUTION Laser Surgery
Class IV Laser
Safety Glasses Required**

Figure 4.1
Protective Eye Wear

With the CO_2 laser, in the invisible wavelength of 10, 600 nm, the use of clear plastic eye protection is recommendable. The use of individual glasses is acceptable, although attachable side shields should be used. **Note; contact lenses and 1/2 glasses aren't enough eye protection as the sclera stays exposed.** Eye protection having an optical density of 5-6 (look amber) is needed for Argon wavelengths. Optical density of 6-14 (look green) is needed for Nd: YAG laser wavelengths. For Tunable Dye lasers the glasses worn will depend on the wavelength chosen. When using the Argon and YAG lasers through endoscopes laser irradiation must be attenuated with protective filter caps used on the endoscopes viewing lens. These filters are available from the laser companies or the manufacturer of the endoscopic equipment.

Laser safety procedures should include criteria that describe the use of eye protection for each laser. The rules are monitored by the LSO, and all personnel in the operating room are required to wear protective eyewear. The American National Standards Institute recommends that those persons who will be routinely exposed to laser irradiation, for medical/legal reasons, have proper examinations to determine baseline medical data. The requirements of this examination would fulfill risk management criteria, preventing a potential workman's

compensation litigation. The medical examination should include:
- visible acuity examination with fundus pictures
- medical history including;
  - ocular and dermatologic systems
  - history of medication, especially those that may be photosensitizing
  - examination of various eye structures about the type of wavelength produced by the laser systems being used

Each facility should establish criteria for frequency of the medical examinations. The first examination should be preformed before participation in laser treatments. Periodic examinations should follow any suspected laser injury and before termination of employment.

The nurse, as the patient's advocate, during surgical intervention, with the laser must consider the patient's safety. If the patient is under general anaesthetic his/her eye should be covered when using the CO_2 with moist gauze pads and taped closed or protective eye shields used, for YAG, a green towel or non-reflective aluminum foil eye shields used. If the operative procedure is under local anesthesia, the patient must wear eye protection of the correct optical for the laser wavelength being used. The patient should be given an explanation regarding wearing eye protection before their surgical procedure. Patient education shouldn't only include safety but all aspects of the laser procedure to include the risks and potential outcomes of the laser treatment. Documentation of all safety measures taken during the procedure should be recorded in the nurses' notes or on the laser log. (see the Appendix)

As laser systems are a complex medical device with electronic, optical, cooling systems and high power electrical requirements, the Biomedical Departments must become involved during the early acquisition process. Another safety consideration when using the laser is electrical hazards. All equipment used in the operating room and other patient care area in health care facilities must follow codes established by the American National Standard Electrical Code. The installation of each laser must follow the manufacturer's recommendations insuring proper electrical circuits and grounding requirements. It's advisable to dedicate a circuit in each operating room, treatment room or clinical area for laser use only. All installation requirements are specified and should be followed exactly to prevent product liability by the manu-

Laser Safety

facturer. Should special requirements be identified, enough time needs to be projected for completion of renovation. Specific requirements to be identified are:

1. Electrical type, in volts and amperes needed to operate each laser used in the area.
   a. this may need isolated panels being installed.
2. If water is a needed utility the pressure and place must be specified.
3. Self contained lasers may give off an increased amount of heat. The air exchanges in the area of in stallation should be checked to determine exchanges and cubic foot units of flow determined.

Fire is another potential hazard during laser use. When prepping the patient before making the surgical incision the prep solution should be non flammable products. Most prep solutions have limited amounts of a flammable ingredient, however, to avoid ignition it's best to have a dry site. Solutions other than those used to prepare the surgical field that may be used during a laser procedure are; **Lugols, Schillers, Acetic Acid, and Toludine Blue,** these areas must be dry, also.

Flammable products such as **alcohol** or **acetone** should **never** be used. Drapes used during operative procedures, whether they're of a nonwoven or cloth material, are subject to ignition or vaporization when directly exposed to the laser beam. The use of surgical incise drapes (plastic) is to avoided if the laser will be used. To avoid this hazard the use of laser barrier constructed material on the areas around the surgical incision can be or should be draped with wet towels when using the CO_2 laser, the other lasers don't need a barrier. However, when using the Nd: YAG laser green towels would afford some barrier. The tissue surrounding the operative site should be packed with wet gauze packs, sponges or cottonoids can be used in the oropharynx during CO_2 laser procedures. These sponges must be kept wet during the whole procedure to avoid combustion.

To avoid inadvertent firing of the laser, the unit should be switched to a standby mode, when the surgeon isn't using the instrument. Because the laser is activated by a foot switch, to avoid confusion when an electro-cautery is being used simultaneously, a hand-trol is recommended, or the electro-cautery foot switch should be placed for the assistant to operate.

Anesthesia safety is paramount when using the laser during aerodigestive or oropharynx surgical procedures. When using the CO/2 laser for procedures in the oral airway the anaesthetic agents should be non-flammable, have rapid induction, smooth recovery and early return to airway reflexes. It's essential that the vocal cords are immobile during the procedure. Muscle relaxants are used during surgery, preventing inadvertent movements of the patient during laryngeal laser procedures. Care should be exercised to avoid sudden movement of the patient or operating room table during the procedure.

The endotracheal tube recommended for use during surgery has been the red rubber tube wrapped with aluminum foil tape, but recently, laser shielded tubes have been introduced by several manufacturers. Red rubber and silicone tubes burn with less intensity and have little toxic combustible products. The aluminum tape is wrapped helically, that's distal to proximal with overlap, then proximal to distal again with overlap. Always test the tape before using, confirming the laser beam doesn't penetrate. This method avoids gaping when curved, the use of the tape reflects the laser energy if hit by the beam. Using an endotracheal tube with a balloon, can be filled with normal saline and a drop of methylene blue. If the laser beam would impact the balloon causing rupture, it'd immediately be evident as the methylene blue would "bleed" on the cottoniod pack around the tube, also, a "heat sink" effect happens and decreases potential ignition. The use of polyvinylcholoride endotracheal tubes **shouldn't** be used in the presence of oxygen, as it supports combustion and the endotracheal tube will ignite making not only fire, but toxic fumes. Post operative complications are critical and cause long-term respiratory problems.

Venturi or jet ventilation anesthesia can be used as an alternative to endotracheal anesthesia during intra-oral and aerodigestive procedures. An advantage of this approach is that it allows the physician clear viewing of the lesion without working around the endotracheal tube. There's a flexible metal endotracheal tube available, the balloon must be manually attached. One problem with this method is that the balloon when inflated isn't symmetrical and can potentially cause trauma to the trachea. Manufacturers are beginning to research other materials for endotracheal tubes that are appropriate for a variety of laser wavelengths.

Other hazards can be: second and third degree burns from incidental direct beam interaction on tissue. These burns first have immediate pain response and healing is usually good with no re-occurring infection. These burns are treated conventionally. Another problem can be ignition of methane gas being expelled by the patient while

Laser Safety

lasing in the perianal area or in the colon. When lasing in the perianal area, if unable to empty the bowel, placing a wet gauze, cotton ball or using a tampon in the lower rectum can absorb the gas and prevent burns. For colo-rectal laser treatments the use of the Nd: YAG laser with coaxial saline prevents the ignition of gases that may be trapped in the colon.

Using the Nd; YAG laser during a fiberoptic endoscopic procedure the anesthesiologist and physician must be aware the same combustible hazards exist, The potential combustible hazards are increased because the coating on the fiber bundle may also be ignited. The same anaesthetic precautions should be followed when using YAG in the oral or aerodigestive tract, as when using the CO2 laser. Another recommendation to prevent further ignition of the fiberoptic bundle is to have the manufacturer install a laser protected tip on the endoscopes used for laser surgery. The porcelain or ebonized tip reduces laser reflection preventing possible ignition of the tip of the fiber bundle.

The physician must have a clear field of operation to safely use the laser verifying the laser fiber tip has sufficiently cleared the end of the fiberscope, the use of video equipment help in being able to document this event. Should the tip not exit the scope with enough length the laser energy fragments the fiber bundle and makes in unusable. In non-contact laser surgery the fiber must be kept clean for proper delivery of the energy to the target tissue. Should the fiber touch tissue it would burn the quartz tip and must be removed. Another fiber must be attached to the delivery system to resume the procedure. The burnt fiber tip will need to be repaired before in can be reused.

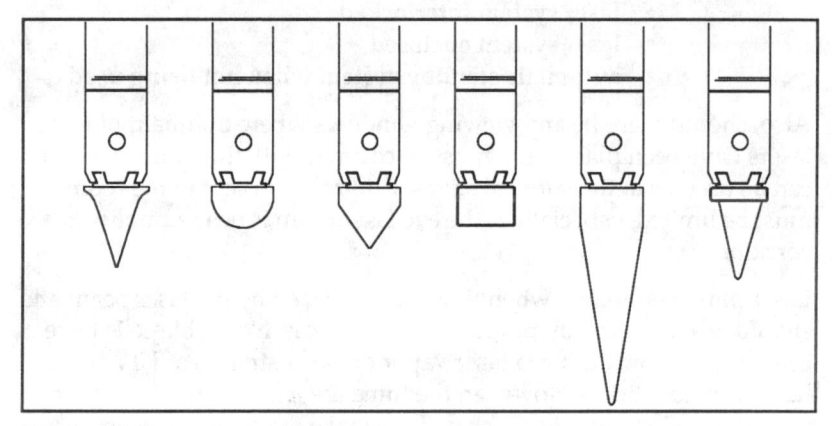

Figure 4.2
Synthetic Sapphire Probes and Scalpels

The sapphire quartz contact probes and scalpels are designed to use with the YAG laser in contact with tissue. These probes are connected to the fibers with a universal couple or come with disposable/reusable fibers, and don't need reprepping for continued use.

Safe use of laser retinal photocoagulators is another concern. Although these laser emit less optical power, the are still a Class 4 laser. Most optical lasers use a slit lamp bio-microscope to deliver a variable cone of radiation through the cornea. Although the beam power used is very low, usually less than 0.5 watts, it still represents a serious eye hazard if misdirected. A collimated beam striking a clear cornea could provide a sharp cone of back reflection. Manufacturers have designed most optic delivery systems so a reflected beam from the cornea is stopped by the instrument itself. If a gonioscopic contact lens is being used, hazardous reflected beams can be deflected at any angle and may pass through the openings in some instruments. All personnel, except the ophthalmologist viewing the eye should wear proper eye protection.

The introduction of the pulsed Nd: YAG laser to ophthalmology presents increased awareness for laser safety either in the physicians office or eye clinic. All staff or other personnel, except the patient and physician, must wear eye protection of the proper optical density. The physician is protected from incidental beam reflection as there's an automatic attenuator built into the laser that drops to protect his/her eyes as the laser is fired. Safety precautions when using the mode-locked or Q-switched YAG ophthalmological lasers, new to health care, are:

- **use of attenuated filters**
- **laser system interlocked**
- **laser system enclosed**
- **automatic standby system when not being used**

Also, should there be any viewing windows where ophthalmologic lasers have been placed, the must be covered with the same material can be used as in the surgical suites. Controlled access to the room must be limited, especially if the eye laser room is near a public corridor.

Laser plume is created when tissue is vaporized by the laser beam and should be evacuated by proper suction devices. No viable cells have been grown from cultured laser vapor or DNA strands of HIV virus have been identified. However, the fume are noxious and can cause nausea, vomiting and headaches. The smoke evacuation system should include a humidity filter to remove steam from vaporized

Laser Safety

water, filters to remove particulate matter and have an optional deodorizing feature. The hospital central vacuum system isn't designed to handle a high volume of laser plume. If the internal suction system is being used for minor procedures, a disposable filter device should be installed between the wall manifold and suction cannister. This filter prevents particulate matter from entering the internal vacuum system and should be changed after each operating day.

If the smoke evacuator has been used on a viral disease such as; condyloma, AID's or herpes, the disposable items should be discarded following the contaminated case procedure. Laser plume limits visibility during endoscopic procedures. New laser filter valves are available to incorporate into the suction system to evacuate smoke without losing wither coaxial gases or pneumoperitonium.

For continued safe practice when using the laser a pre-and post-procedure checklist will assure proper operation of the equipment and begins preventive maintenance. This checklist is the responsibility of the laser specialists who has received special training in laser safety and maintenance. The laser check out procedure is done each day before laser procedures begin and if the laser has been moved long distances, this checking procedure should be documented. If the laser is moved room-to-room frequently, the check-out procedure may need to be done more often. If a problem is noted, the physician and operating room supervisor are notified, immediately. If necessary, the biomedical technician or department should be notified, and may be able to intervene and resolve the problem. The laser check list should include:

1. Keys available.
2. Handpieces, micromanipulator, and accessories available and sterile, as needed.
3. Laser gas levels correct (as necessary), and regulars are working properly.
4. Laser has electrical power.
5. Laser works in all modes.
6. The laser beam has coaxial alignment with the HeNe beam.
7. Foot switch works properly.
8. Microprocessor or power controls working.
9. Stand-by mode works.

The check list should be signed by the person completing the process. For continued proper use of the laser, all handpieces and accessories must be handled with care, cleaned properly after each uses and carefully stored, in the proper containers.

The lens of the handpieces must **never** be sterilized under steam and pressure. The special coating on the lens will crack and there will be significant reduction of laser energy and beam divergence. These lens must be replaced should this incident happen. When cleaning the micromanipulator the gimbled mirror that directs the laser beam shouldn't be touched and only cleaned with lens paper, contact lens used with ophthalmology lasers must be inspected for "pitting" when being cleaned, as the "pitted" lens can cause incidental beam reflections.

Each laser procedure should be properly documented to provide clinical information, records for governmental inspection, as needed, and medical/legal safeguards. For continued insurance of proper and safe use of lasers in medicine and surgery, approved policies and procedures must be established. Each facility must develop its own standard operating procedures to provide safety to patients and personnel, optimum use, and proper care of each laser. A variance report is done and send to Risk Management and the Laser Committee should an incident happen, the report should be reviewed and recommendations made to rectify the occurrence. Also, the Laser Committee must keep current on future laser indications and applications. As new laser are introduced, additions or addendum may need to be made to existing safety rules and policies and procedures.

SUMMARY

Lasers are capable of concentrating high energy outputs into small, collimated beam, potentially; this could be dangerous. Laser use and safety fall under the jurisdiction of several governmental agencies and care classified as medical devices. Lasers are a Class III medical device and a Class 4, subclassification. The laser used in medicine are a Class 4 laser with established safety guidelines.

For safe patient and personnel use, each facility must establish approved safety criteria. This criteria should include; medical staff privilege and credentialing criteria, appointment of a laser safety officer, and standard operating policies and procedures.

When renovation of the laser therapy treatment area is considered, physical safety and building codes are important to ensure safe practice, to include covering the viewing windows and controlled access to the areas where lasers are being used.

Intra-operative safety policies and procedures should be defined, considering; proper eye protection, surgical instrumentation, use of prep solutions and draping material, anesthesia precautions, smoke and fire hazards and proper operation of the laser equipment.

Personnel policy should be established for medical evaluation, particularly ophthalmologic and dermatologic examinations of laser users to establish a baseline before employment and laser usage.

The future of laser therapy lies with the user, and it's imperative for the safety of the patients, physicians and other medical personnel that all understand each laser regarding its safe use in medical applications.

Part 2
Laser Program Development

CHAPTER 5
HOW TO DECIDE

The laser, like all technology acquires its value only through proper use. The goal of each health care facility is to provide responsible delivery of this care. A laser program has a basis for economical viability they are:

- Inpatient procedures are performed more efficietly, generally reducing operating room time and anesthesia time, reducing length of stay.
- The impact on the DRG's relates to several factors;
  - Short term DRG's turn into out-patients
  - Less consumables used
  - Reduces need for multiple transfusions
  - Keeps the patient in the community
  - Increases Ambulatory Care patient population
  - Is a good marketing tool for the facility

With the technological advances in medicine spanning basic research, diagnostic capabilities, minimally invasive procedures and therapeutic tools, health care providers must make creative decisions for the delivery of quality care. When considering the acquisition of laser systems many factors must be considered. Laser systems represent a capital investment, subsequently, an organized approach to implementation is necessary to develop an effectively used program.

Feasibility studies to assess needs begins with a medical staff survey and includes their existing practice trends, expected referral patterns and patient mix. Furthermore, a cost analysis is done, potential utilization reviewed, space allocation and installations costs budgeted, procurement methods decided, staff education including physicians and nurses planned, governmental regulations reviewed, program trend analysis format designed, and marketing techniques explored. When the study is complete and the analysis shows that a laser program would be a viable strategic goal, the next step is the appointment of a group of people to plan and implement the program. A multi-specialty laser committee is appointed by administration with the approval of the President of the Medical Staff.

This committee serves as a nucleus providing medical leadership for the program. Members of the committee are physicians with interest and intent to use lasers in their practice to include anesthesiology. Other representatives are from administration; operating room services, nursing services, quality assurance and the biomedical departments.

The purpose, goals and objectives of the committee are well defined, and functional reports are presented to the Executive Committee monthly. The laser committee is to coordinate those activities into an organized program for medical and surgical specialties. The aim of this committee, with change, as the program develops, should incorporate the following goals and should be attainable by this group:

- Monitoring and evaluating all activities related to the laser program.
- Recommendation of educational criteria, to meet the credentialing mechanism at the facility.
- Educate physicians, nurses and other personnel in the use of the laser.
- Establish quality assurance criteria.
- Develop a preceptor program or continuing educa tion process.
- Recommendation of laser equipment and accessories for procurement.
- Recommendation of standards of practice for use of lasers and laser safety.
- Develop a mechanism to assess the trends of the program to justify expansion.

The laser committee's activities evolve to meet the facilities established strategic goals.

The first responsibility is to survey the medical staff to get commitment, with intent to use and a define a projected patient population, to evaluate the type of laser needed to meet their needs. The survey involves the medical staff in the development of the program, and provides early input for decisions in the acquisition process. Based on the results of the survey, commitment by physicians and administration, the committee can review and recommend specific laser equipment. It's proper for the committee to have the laser manufacturers make a presentation to determine the type of laser being purchased. There are several considerations in acquiring a laser:

- Type of laser, buy the state of the art. Technology is changing so rapidly it's essential to buy the most advanced system or one that can be retrofitted to meet the changing needs of multi-disciplined use.

- Mobility increases usage. Most laser systems are mobile and must be moved with care and technical aid.

- Training and continued education of physicians and support personnel is important to maintain a viable program.

- Service commitment is a prime factor when choosing a laser as down time is frustrating and costly.

An evaluation process should be developed so the primary and potential secondary users can have access to the equipment. The evaluation program is a well developed process with documentation by each physician and a summary developed for an administrative decision for proper laser acquisition based on the criteria establish for utilization. Most health care facilities have evaluation forms and summary sheets used when capital equipment is purchased.

It may be necessary to develop a presentation to the Administrative Council and the Board of Trustees, before final approval for purchase is confirmed. Programmatic goals should be addressed and primary goals of the program planned being implemented expediently, meeting the strategic goals of the organization.

Establishing educational criteria and recommended standards for practice for laser use is another charge to the committee, Although laser privileges for individual physicians using laser is reviewed departmentally, the laser committee is responsible for establishing the basic criteria. Educational criteria that's established must be realistic, attainable and functional for each facility. The basis for the criteria is for standard practice and laser safety. A recommended criterion could be:

> **The completion of a Category I, Continuing Medical ducation Program (12-16 hours) that includes didactic and clinical application of lasers in medicine and surgery.** A preceptorship can be incorporated into the cedentialing mechanism with documentation of a certificate, kept intra-departmentally or with the medical staff office.

The Joint Commission on Accreditation for Hospitals has developed guidelines for physicians and is suggesting that other health care provides should be credentialed. Their guidelines recommend "a process designed to assure that all individuals who provide patient care services...are competent to provide such service. The quality of patient care services provided by these individuals is reviewed as part of the hospitals quality assurance program."

Continued education of physicians, nurses, and support staff is implemented and monitored by the laser committee. Many manufacturers will help in the early education of physicians and support staff, but for the maintenance of safe practice, continuing education is important. There are many established, certified, on-going physician education programs in disciplines, readily available today. Several schools with curricula in laser technology have been established across the country. Training programs for nursing personnel have been established, many of them by state approved nursing organizations, for continued educations credits. All training programs should be conducted in a setting conducive to learning. Another way to maintain continuing education is to develop seminars or workshops being sponsored by the hospital's education department. All programs developed should try to meet the learners needs. Physicians must understand all aspects of photobiological interactions of lasers on tissue, and the application of the various wavelengths in their specialty. The physicians program should include animate clinical laboratory experience. All laser programs sponsored by the facility should be reviewed by the laser committee.

A major responsibility of the laser committee is develop, review, recommend and implement policies and procedures. Laser safety rules are approved and monitored by the laser safety officer. As the multi-use laser program develops, policies and procedures are updated and are reviewed by the committee on a continuing basis. Several policies and procedures are recommended being approved and established with and before the early start-up of the program. These are:
1. Purpose and function of the laser committee.
2. Physician education and privilege criteria.
3. Education of laser personnel.
4. Laser safety rules.
5. Set-up and operational procedures.
6. Laser maintenance and documentation.
7. Documentation of laser procedures.
8. Laser charges.
9. Occurrence or variance reporting criteria.
10. Quality Assurance criteria.
11. Approval of new procedures if their clinical efficacy is recognized.

As each program develops and expands, the policy and procedure manual must be updated, added and reviewed on an on-going basis.

The laser committee has extended responsibility for recommending personnel to operate an efficient multi-use laser program. Should the hospital become involved in research or investigational studies, protocols must be defined, reviewed and approved by the Institutional Review Board. If the hospital doesn't have this body in place, the laser committee can assume the responsibility for review and approval. Many lasers are still considered investigational. There's considerable research being done with varying wavelengths of YAG, Excimer, and Tunable Dye lasers, and the clinical efficacy of the lasers systems haven't been totally established, yet.

The manufacturers and/or distributors of these lasers will help the physician, Laser Committee and Institutional Review Board with F.D.A. approval or the development of protocols being presented to the Investigational Review Board.

Tunable Dye Lasers used in Photodynamic Therapy are considered investigational in the United States are subject to the Food and Drug Administration's regulations. All procedures done with these lasers must have approved protocols with designated principal investigators. Each protocol describes in detail the procedure, method, evaluation and follow-up mechanism. The principal investigators sign an agreement with the laser company to follow the established protocol, complete all necessary paper work, submit summaries for periodic review by the laser company and the F.D.A. When participating in a project with the investigational lasers, a special consent form must be used. The consent includes a description of the procedure and all the risks in it, and must be signed by the patient and certified by the physician doing the laser treatment. Institutions participating in laser treatments with investigational devices are subject to review by the F.D.A. All laser patient charts and other documentation is reviewed for compliance and accuracy. It's the principal investigator's responsibility to monitor all activities regarding the approved laser treatment protocol.

As other lasers currently being used in clinical applications of medicine and surgery aren't considered investigational, consent for laser treatment should be incorporated into the surgical procedure consent forms currently used by most health care facilities.

For medical/legal considerations all patients having laser treatments must have informed consent to include the risks and potential outcomes of their procedure.

With the fundamentals of a multi-use laser program established and approved by the Medical Executive Committee, Hospital Administration and Board of Trustees, procurement and installation of laser systems, choice of support personnel, physician and nurse education, the implementation of laser treatment practice in the hospital is ready to begin.

SUMMARY

There's a predictable growth in the medical laser industry of about 26% a year until the next century. With the proliferation of laser technology in medicine and surgery today, how do you decide if a laser program is a viable strategic goal for your institution?

A feasibility study surveys the medical staff for commitment and intent to use, and a projected population, should be finished. The survey results are evaluated and analyzed for cost effectiveness, program utilization, budgetary effect, commitment by the medical staff and long range viability for corporate commitment of the program.

The laser committee or task force should be appointed as a nucleus for recommendation of equipment, development of educational criteria, implementation of policies and procedures, to establish safety rules, monitor investigational programs, and participate in continued education of physician and support staff.

The Laser Committee reports directly to the Medical Executive Committee for support and direction of the laser program.

CHAPTER 6
PROCUREMENT AND INSTALLATION OF LASERS

There are approximately 25 major medical laser manufacturers in the industry today. Each manufacturer offers various options both in laser equipment, accessories, education, service and procurement methods. The expectation each health care facility has, is that the vendors will make a comprehensive presentation to include:

- Over view of the state of the art, especially the features of this manufacturer's laser systems.
- A description of accessories required and available to use the laser in the treatment modalities expected to be performed at the facility.
- Education support of physicians, nurses, and staff support.
- Details of warranty and service contracts for each laser.
- Manufacturer History.
- Detailed user list.
- Installation requirements.

Most laser manufacturers will negotiate with the facility for many added features to meet their needs.

Additional provisions may include general in-service programs for all medical and nursing staff, and technical schooling for biomedical personnel; other contractual services from the company could include laser technicians or nursing personnel on-site for a specified period of time, for start-up support. All service agreements should be reviewed by the hospital attorney, making sure monetary reimbursement and guaranteed turn-around-time are specifically delineated. However, should the biomedical personnel of the facility attend the service school, points of service can be negotiated to reduce the total contract cost.

There are several steps in the acquisition process that should precede procurement. These steps are:

- Identifying the type and power of the laser systems needed to meet the needs of the facility.
- Identify the laser companies that sell those particular types of lasers.

Procurement and Installation of Lasers

- Send letters to the manufacturers with general specifications requesting bids for consideration, with a time limit for return of information.
- Identify to the vendors the contact person(s) at the facility.
- After all the bids have been received and reviewed anevaluation process should be developed.

Why should the facility go through this process? Each laser, although may be the same wavelength, has different features that the physician must choose for his practice techniques. The evaluation process should be developed and controlled by the facility and laser coordinator. Several elements in the process should be considered:

1. The development of a simple survey document to be completed by the potential users, to include the nursing personnel that will be involved.
2. Site selection for demonstration that provides easy access for the physician. A recommended site may be the isolation room in the recovery room.
3. Notification sent to the physicians regarding time, place and their responsibility in assisting in the decision making process.
4. The evaluation and demonstration of the lasers should **not** occur simultaneously as that dilutes the ability to concentrate on the specific features of the systems.
5. The evaluation process should not take more than two to three days per laser compant and completed in a specified length of time.
6. The summary documented should be prepared as a side by side comparison. This document can be re viewed and presented for decision making.

When considering the purchase of Ophthalmic laser there are several features to evaluate that are different from lasers used for surgical procedures, they are:

- The *delivery system,* such as the slit lamps are used to target the laser energy to the desired intra-ocular structure. The laser should not be incorporated into the slit lamp in such a way that it hampers the action of the slit lamp. The laser should have high optical resolution with unimpededviewing optics.

- The *aiming system* should provide a range of intensities that are required by different tissue targets.
- The *ergonomics* of the system, such as work space, storage for lens, ability to adjust the laser light and adjustable chairs for the comfort of the physician and patient should be considered. Visible read out displays that are legible or that are incorporated inthe optics are most efficient. The firing controls whether hand or foot are a matter of individual preference.

On completion of the evaluation process a purchase order is "cut", this should document all elements of the purchase. These are:

- Total price with all accessories itemized to include the prices as a replacement budget may need to be developed.
- All accessories, i.e., endoscopes, glasses, smoke evacuators and their listed prices. (these can be ordered from other companies, sometimes at lower cost)
- What inservice includes, and when and whether or not it is repeatable, as needed. If not at what cost to the facility can it be repeated.
- All technical service schools or other biomedical training has been identified.
- Any discount identified.
- Make sure service and educational manuals will be included.
- The availability of service and guaranteed onsite time for service, to include facility responsibility for the onsite visit.
- Availability of technician or nursing personnel for initial start-up procedures.
- Ongoing responsibility and who or what the company or distributor provides should be defined.
- Installation requirements outline in full detail.
- Delivery date guaranteed.
- Any potential up-grades or retrofits that occur in thenear future and who assumes the responsibility for these changes.

Procurement and Installation of Lasers

When all presentations have been made and the recommendations submitted, actual procurement of the laser and related accessories is the next step in the implementation of a laser program. Several financial methods are available to health care facilities:

1. Out right purchase, is the most advantageous to the vendor and the facility. The facility has immediate capitalization an depreciation of the equipment and the manufacturer has his payment in accordance with established terms.

2. Lease/purchase is possible through the manufacturer, with higher interest rates, or through the hospital's leasing company with a a lower interest rate available. Leasing has an advantage of fast amortization and a option to purchase at the end of the contract or to exchange the equipment for newer, updated technology.

3. Some laser distribution companies will consider placing laser for a usage fee. The laser is installed with an agreement of a guaranteed usage per month. The hospital pays the company a fixed price per use. If the laser is used more frequently than the fixed price, the laser company makes a profit. If the laser is not used at the guaranteed rate, the hospital must pay the fixed user price often not reimbursable and the laser distributor has the option to with draw the laser from the institution, as agreed. A usage fee arrangement may seem a viable option, especially in current cost containment efforts inthe industry. An other option for consideration in this method of procurement is to have a percentage of the usage fee go toward the purchase of the laser in an agreed time commitment. The advantage of this agreement would be the opportunity to evaluate the usage of the laser in the physician's practice, to determine its viability to a multi-use concept.

4. A physician may agree to purchase the laser for the institution and establish a reimbursement mechanism for payment of the laser. A contractual agreement delineating use, maintenance responsibilities and invoicing is signed by both parties. Advantages

of this method of procurement are; physician commitment to use, release from the initial financial responsibility, and a potential tax shelter option for the physician.

5. A group of physician may want to establish a joint venture with the facility. This would provide the money for the equipment, and a lease agreement can be contracted with the hospital for use, with reimbursement dollars defined in the contract. The physicians would invoice the usage fee and be paid by the hospital. There are not as many advantages of this method as the tax laws have been revised, however, there is immediate cash for purchase of equipment and physician commitment to the use of the laser.

For a multi-laser facility, the ability to use the various methods of creative financing may be important to the continued viability of the laser program. Most lasers have accessories that are needed to deliver the laser beam to the appropriate tissue. These accessories are; handpieces, with different focal lengths, with an assortment of mirror attachments, fibers of various types and lengths, fiber polishing kits, micromanipulators for connection to the microscope, regulators and gas tanks. Other associated accessories are; smoke evacuators systems, proper signs, drapes for the laser, instrumentation, and proper eye protection. For the various specialities there will be specific accessories that will need to be considered, they are; endoscopes, both rigid and flexible, and catheters for some of the newer procedures. Newer accessories are available for the Nd:YAG laser that enables the surgeon to perform contact laser procedures, they are contact probes and scalpels. Its is advantageous to purchase accessories from various manufacturers that specialize in this equipment.

LASER ACCESSORIES

Lasers must have an optical interface for delivery of the laser beam to the target of impact. Each laser has a variety of accessories available:

Carbon Dioxide lasers can be used with hand-held equipment or connected to a microscope. The accessories available for the CO_2 laser are handpieces with a variety of angles and focal lengths, regulators for the CO_2 gas tanks and tanks of premixed gas. The microscope connection, a mechanical micromanipulator is available with a variable lens adjusting system to match the focal length of the lens

Procurement and Installation of Lasers

system on the microscope. The other accessories are rigid bronchoscopes, laproscopes, cystoscopes, and newly developed arthroscopes for large and small joint evaluation. Several instrument manufacturers have developed special laser instruments that are available in anodized or matte finish. Other accessories such as; quartz or titanium rods or laser mirrors will need to be available for some of the procedures. The sealed tube CO2 lasers will not require regulators or gas tanks as the CO2 gas is contained and a catalyst mixed to re-bond the molecules for continued use is a sealed system that will need refilling approximately every three-five years, depending on use. Smoke evacuators must be available for CO_2 and YAG lasers. Laser plume filters are available for in-line evacuation through the central vacuum system, when procedures are done that produce limited plume.

Continuous Wave Nd:YAG lasers are used with flexible endoscopes and can be use free hand with a special handpiece adaptor. The various fiber delivery systems are available for esophageal, bronchial, laryngeal, gastric and urologic work. These fiber systems are used with the appropriate endoscope. Other accessories that are needed when the YAG laser is used with endoscopes are attenators that cover the eye pieces of the scope of the correct optical density.

A new, revolutionary accessory for the Nd:AYG laser is the synthetic sapphire ceramic probes and scalpels. Because these particularly shaped probes and scalpels are made of special ceramic material, they concentrate all the energy at the tip, and they use less total energy. Subsequently, the power output is reduced below 40 watts and you can touch tissue with no detrimental effects to the tip and/or fiber.

The use of these new ceramics with its various geometrical shapes reduces the thermal zone of necrosis and can cut and coagulate, simultaneously. Telfon clad or bare fibers are still used for a variety of procedures and can be burned or broken easily. A fiber polishing kit is available for purchase and a nurse or biomedical technician can be taught how to repair them. It is not economical to return them to the company for repair.

The *Argon and Nd:YAG* ophthalmic lasers require the purchase of special gonioscopic lenses to be used during the procedure. The air-cooled 5 watt Argon laser that is available and can be used for Plastic and Dermatological surgery has a collimated handpiece for a delivery system. There is special eye protection, a stainless steel "eye-cup", to be inserted over the cornea during these types of procedures when done on or around the eyelid.

The Tunable Dye and other visible laser wavelengths are used with a fiber delivery system and the fibers must must be cut and polished often, The same fiber polishing kit bought for YAG laser fibers can be used and the same techniques for polishing employed. Also, the cylindrical diffusers that are used during these procedures must be handled with care.

INSTALLATION

Each laser type has specific requirements for installation. However, the first requirement is to determine usage and appropriate space for installation. If the laser will have miltidiscipline use there should be guideline established as to scheduling priorities and whether the laser should be moved from a pre-determined location to another department for expanded use. The revised ANSI Z136.3 guidelines suggest that, "if the laser is to be used in a controlled well trafficked area, an door lock is recommended for safety." However, these new guideline will leave the issue of "inter-locks" to the discretion of the Laser Safety Officer. The types of locks, if necessary should be from the inside of the room and "panic" hardware can be used.

Most medical lasers are mobile with exception of those that require a fixed water source for cooling such as the Argon lasers used in Ophthalmology. In renovation of space for laser installation several items must be considered:

- Space Required
- Multi use
- Electrical circuits
- Need for water access including drainage
- Window viewing protection
- Controlled access

Some of the medical laser are bulky equipment weighing up to 850 pounds. The lasers are heavy with resonating cavities and articulated arms that make them difficult to move great distances.

To develop increase laser use, the equipment must be readily available to each surgical and some medical disciplines. The engineering and biomedical departments should assist in determining the installation of electrical and water outlets, as necessary. Also, the facilities engineering departments will know the required electrical codes for the state and city. Also, they will be acquainted whether any other testing of the equipment may be required before it is put into use.

Procurement and Installation of Lasers

The CO2 laser power requirements range from 115 volts, 15 amperes to 220 volts, and 30 amperes. The power output form the CO2 laser is 1-100 watts. No special wiring is required as they are self contained units with there awn water or air cooling devices. However, these lasers often have two outlets to handle the larger electrical limits, and isolated power transformers may be necessary. It is recommended that the lasers have a dedicated electrical circuit to protect it from possible power shut-downs from overloading the circuit. The laser should be on the emergency power circuit.

The YAG laser have different requirements for installation, and have power outputs from 1-150 watts, several types of YAG laser must have recirculating external water supply and available to a drain source. The electrical requirements may be 208 three phase, 30 amperes for electricity. The YAG laser for ophthalmology has other requirements; electricity 110 to 115 volts, 15 amperes or 440 volts with 40 amperes and can be cooled by external water or recirculating room air. There are several space requirements of the ophthalmologic lasers.

The large Argon ophthalmic laser must dissipate heat generated, the the Argon-ion laser tubes must be water cooled. The water flow should be 2.5 to 5.0 gallons per minute with a drain source available. Power requirements may vary by manufacturer, but generally range between 190-240 volts, 3 phase with 40 amperes per phase. There is a three phase input transformer available to accept phase voltages between 190-240 volts.

The smaller, mobile Argon lasers that can be used for ophthalmology but usually used on Dermato-Plastics work on 110-120 volts, 30 amperes cooled by ambient air and moves easily from place to place. There are other mobile Argon lasers with Krypton but, require a external water source for cooling, these are connected with a "quick disconnect" valve.

The newer Tunable Dye laser for ophthalmology have other considerations to include changing of the dyes used and disposable of these waste products.

The ophthalmic laser, Argon and YAG, require a slit lamp as part of their laser beam delivery system. Most manufacturers include the slit lamp with the laser console, although the slit lamp can be an optional accessory.

The Tunable Dye lasers, use in photodynamic therapy are immobile, large lasers that require extensive installation considerations. The laser should be installed with accessibility to an operating room for both inpatient and outpatient use.

Space requirements are approximately 10 feet by 10 beet with sufficient air-flow as this laser generates heat. The laser weighs approximately 485 pounds. The power requirements vary with manufacturer but, generally you need 440 volts, 30 amperes of electricity, plus water and a drain source immediately available. The water pressure is at 50 pounds per square inch, with a flow rate of 5.0 gallons per minute. The may require a booster pump at the water source to avoid any decrease or fluctuation that may occur in the facilities water pressure, as it would immediately activate the lasers safety features and shut it down. There is a dye laser connected to the main laser source that usually has a 10-20 watt output. A mechanism for disposal must be readily available, a sink with a special trap installed in or near the laser room. Another installation requirement for the Tunable Dye laser is a "pass-through" for the fiber delivery system to reach the patient during his/her laser treatment.

As described most lasers vary in size from small, about 125 pounds to large, unwieldy, and heavy about 850 pounds pieces of equipment. To know where to use, palace and possibly store this equipment will take prior planning. Although, the lasers are considered a somewhat delicate tool, the do have to be locked in a store room or closet, as the keys should be controlled by the laser nurse or safety officer. It is important that the users all acquire a knowledge and understanding of how to move and care for the lasers, appropriately.

If lasers are to be moved from place to place on the same level, two persons should be involved, especially when moving the CO_2 laser. The articulated arm must not be bumped or the mirrors any mis-align. The floors should be smooth and care must be taken when moving across the expansion joints. Engineering departments can assist by placing a rubber core over the expansion joint for smooth transition across the floor.

Laser do give off some heat through dissipation of the photon through the resonating cavity and are either water or air cooled. In a small operating room or treatment room there should be enough air exchanges to keep the room at comfortable temperature.

SUMMARY

There are a multitude of laser companies in the market place, today and the procurement of lasers are negotiable. The purchasing agent must know the vendor's responsibilities for presentation and evaluation. the evaluation process is important so the laser selected will have the highest usage possible to be cost effective. Creative financing is an important concept when developing a multi- use strategies. All associated laser accessaries must be identified during the purchasing process.

Other contractual agreements, such as; education for staff ,service contracts, technical school for the biomedical personnel and company laser field representative available, as needed by the facility, for start-up should be included in the initial contractual agreement.

All lasers have specific requirements for installation and should be followed for guarantee of all warranties. The manufacturers will work with the facility's Engineering Department insuring installation.

The purchase of the appropriate accessories needed to perform laser procedures is an important consideration, especially budgetary, for the expanded use of each laser system.

The smallest space should be about 180 square feet, usually this is for the ophthalmic lasers, however, lasers are being placed in the physician's offices and have limited space.

When the Argon and YAG laser are considered for purchase, the electrical and water utilities must be investigated, where the lasers will be used. Contiguous space for multi-use will reduce the cost of renovation and installation.

For outpatient use of the lasers the logistics of patient flow must be considered to expedite the scheduled procedures.

CHAPTER 7
THE ADMINISTRATIVE ROLE

The general corporate strategy of the hospital must be met as new programs are developed for facility planning. As new programs impact on all areas of the facility, administration must choose its strategy for implementation. The success of new programs includes pre-planning, cost analysis, identification of implementation problems, contingency plans to address these problems, and solicitation of cooperation and commitment from all parties involved in the program. Administration improves the chances for success when effective methods is used in laying the ground work to gain commitment and participation of all persons involved with the program.

When a multi-disciplined, multi-laser program is being considered, a feasibility study should be done to analyze all the ramifications of a multi-specialty laser program. The components of the study are:

Physician Commitment must be documented with potential interest to use the acquired laser system. A physician survey is sent to the medical staff with several succinct questions, they are:

- Are you currently using laser in your practice?
- Have you attended any laser education programs?
- If a laser program is implemented would you use the laser?
- What would you expect your patient population for laser usage would be, per month?

Making the survey easy to answer and return for analysis will enhance compliance and completion of the survey form.

Surgical Procedure review must include all areas where procedures are being done; the operating room, outpatient surgery, Gastroenterology Suites, Pulmonary Labs, and Clinics that are managed by the facility. When at least one year's date history of these procedures have been reviewed, assumptions can be made as a conversion factor from conventional procedures to laser procedures and the projected new business that could be created over a define number of years.

Fiscal Responsibilities must be reviewed to include reimbursement class, bad debt allowances, operational costs, and any space renovation costs that may be incurred. These elements are compared to the projected income from the laser procedures. Other components of the financial analysis should include an amortization

The Administrative role

schedule for projected purchases of laser systems, accessories, futures laser purchases, marketing and education costs. Other financial considerations must also be reviewed, with cost conscience providers and consumers, the DRG reimbursements rates should be compared to a cost to charge ratio. A case mix analysis can be reviewed and trends analyzed. This information can be compared to case mix information by physician that will help in the best formula to used to generate the proper charge for the procedure and equipment.

The study report should help with long range planning and physician interest, general cost, and cost effectiveness; including reimbursement, budget, referral patterns, increased utilization of the facility, with implications of new governmental regulations. Other consideration in the development of the program are administrative control, staffing, education, space requirements, installation costs, procurements methods, institutional review board responsibilities, education of physician and nurses and program evaluation. When this study is complete and analysis finished, the program should meet general long range planning and corporate strategic goals before a commitment is made to proceed with program development.

With the commitment to proceed the president of the medical staff or hospital should appoint a task-oriented laser committee to complete the specific program goals. The committee appointed should included physician with high interest in using laser in their practice, and representation from administration, the operating room, nursing, purchasing, and the biomedical department. Other departmental representatives can be added as the program expands. The committee's overall purpose is to evaluate and choose the proper lasers, to developmental education criteria, develop safety rules, policies and procedures, to assist in the continued education of physicians and support staff, and to continually monitor and evaluate the total scope of the program. Letters of intent to use the lasers are sent to the medical staff with a request for projected patient population. This information establishes commitment from the medical staff and the patient information helps in developing the charges for each laser. As the results from the letters are returned, the committee can review the type of lasers that may be needed for the program. From the list of various manufacturers the committee picks specific vendors to make presentations to them as they develop the evaluation process.

The evaluation process includes several components and should be structured, documented, summarized and reviewed for the decision making process. After reviewing the manufacturing list, requesting bids for the proper laser system learned from the feasibility studies, the evaluation process should be planned. The vendors are given a date (s) to bring their system onsite. The laser demonstration area should have easy access for physicians and other personnel involved in the evaluation. An evaluation form developed and completed by each physician, nurse or biomedical personnel. A summary of this information forwarded to the Laser Committee for review and comment, then forwarded to administration for decision and action.

The evaluation form should be easy to complete and should be done when the physician or other personnel participates in the evaluation of the product. The information is a "need to know" is:

- Ease of Use.
- User Friendly Control Panel
- If CO_2, Look at the Balance of the Articulated Arm
- Installation needs and Process
- What Type of Utilities are Needed.
- Power Output Appropriate for Projected Uses.
- What Type of Modes are Available.
- How Easy is it to Set-up.
- What Type of Accessories are Included.
- What is Included in the Education Package.

The summary should include:

- Company, location and history
- Purchase and Operational Costs
- Defined Education Process and repeat inservices
- Technical Support
- Service Agreements
- Accessories and their Cost

After the evaluation process is done, the committee forwards written recommendations to the administration for approval and buy.

For continued safe practice of lasers in medicine and surgery, the Laser Safety Officer (LSO) has the designated responsibility and authority to monitor the laser practice. Specific safety rules are defined, implemented and monitored by the LSO who has the responsibility of discussing any infraction of the rules with the physicians and completing a variance report that's reviewed by the Laser Committee.

The Administrative Role

As an active member of the Laser Committee he/she is involved in the development of policies and procedures, maintains and updates all safety standards, establishes maintenance, repair and documents all service on the lasers. There are many guidelines available through various governmental agencies to establish, specific safety rules for compliance by individual facilities. Approval by the Medical Executive Committee, and Hospital Safety Committee is imperative for medical/legal implications. The procedure of credentialing and continued monitored of safe practice is developed by the committee. The Joint Commission on Accreditation of Hospital guidelines under the chapter of the Governing Body, establish the mechanism of credentialing for privileges granted to practice in the facility.

The guidelines for requesting laser privileges should follow recommended guidelines of the American Society for Lasers Medicine and Surgery:

- Complete a laser privilege form with supporting documentation that meets the credentialing criteria.

- This is reviewed by the Laser Committee and for warded to the Central Credentials Committee for approval and notification forwarded to; requestor, proper administrative personnel, and department chairmen.

- Continued and continuing education must be obtained as new wavelengths are introduced into the facility.

The facility may modify this guideline to meet the medical staff bylaws however, they should include the components outline above.

Policy and procedures are continually being developed as the laser program expands, the Laser Committee is the reviewing and recommending body for the approval process. Recommendations are made by the chairman for approval by the medical executive committee. Policies and procedures that should be developed include those involving:

- Function and purpose of the laser committee.
- Responsibilities of the laser personnel.
- Educational Criteria
- Continuing education process
- Quality Assurance monitoring
- Operational safety
- Occurrence screening and variance reporting mechanisms.

- Set-up and Shut-down procedures.
- Care of equipment and accessories.
- Maintenance schedule.
- Documentation processes
- External monitoring of regulations
- Involvement in Research Projects
- Nursing Responsibilities

The technology of lasers presents concern for administration in medical/legal implications. The policy and procedures help in establishing facility guidelines for standards of practice. Documentation of all laser procedures is important and a laser log or incorporating the laser information in the operative "Nursing Notes" should be kept to include the following information:

- Patient Name and I.D. Number
- Physicians Name, both Surgeon and Referring Physician
- Procedure Performed
- All Safety Precautions Taken
- Type of Anesthesia and Type of Endotracheal Tube used, if necessary
- Energy to Tissue, Mode Changes
- Total time the laser was used
- Any unusual occurrence
- Set-up Check List Signed
- Log signed by laser operator

This information can be useful in a variety of ways; for legal purposes, for review when a follow up procedure is done, quality occurrence monitoring, and for clinical research.

Informed consent, signed by each patient, includes procedure being done and type of laser used. Should investigational protocols be implemented a special operative consent form must be done. These consent forms include statements of risks, and a certification signature of the physician that states "this is informed consent." The Federal Register has published the elements of informed consent that must be incorporated into this document. The Food and Drug Administration has control of investigational lasers and can request to review all data pertinent to this investigation laser any time they elect to review the institutional medical records, the Institutional Review Board can monitor this certification process. When the laser is investigational, the designed principal investigator must work under an approved F.D.A. protocol. The protocols are reviewed by the hospitals institu-

The Administrative Role

tional review board. If the hospital doesn't have this structure, the protocols should be approved by the laser committee. The approved protocol includes a reporting mechanism to the F.D.A. This information gives the F.D.A. feedback regarding the effectiveness of the device and/or treatment.

The cost effectiveness of the program has developed technical nuances with the implementation of DRG's. There's insufficient information about the efficacy of laser treatment, in most specialities, and how it affects the surgical result. The laser is a tool, added to the physicians armamentarium and has been bought by the facility as capital equipment and charges for the use are established. However, a great number of the laser procedures can be done on an outpatient basis and reimbursed on a cost basis. Third party reimbursers have recognized the efficacy of most laser procedures and are paying for them. Many laser codes have been established by the **"Physicians Current Procedures Terminology" (CPT)** for laser reimbursement. DRG grouper programs in the medical records departments cross reference their codes for **ICD-9-CM** reimbursement rates.

Usually, inpatient revenue isn't increased as most laser treated patients have reduced length of stay. The patients recieving photodynamic therapy with the Tunable Dye laser are oncological patients and increased patient days and revenue result from the treatment of these patients. Having a multi-disciplined laser center can increase the referral base of the patient population, based on an aggressive marketing program.

To establish the laser charges, many factors must be considered, including the cost of the laser (s) equipment, accessories, renovation and installation, how long they'll be amortized, and length of depreciation. The patient usage is also a consideration when establishing a flat rate charge for the equipment. A rule of thumb formula is:

$$\frac{\text{Total Cost} \div \text{Years of Amortization}}{\text{Projected patient uses}} \times \% \text{ increase} = \text{Charge}$$

The variable factors are direct and indirect costs and patient population. This can be reviewed each year during the budget process. Another method to establish laser charges would be on an incremental charge based of time of utilization.

Budget is another administrative responsibility. Budget considerations include the following components: (all or some, depending on the

lasers bought)
- Staff
- Service contracts or insurance policies
- Rental or Lease contracts
- CO_2 gas
- Fibers and/or contact probes and scalpels
- Drapes, quartz rods
- Smoke evacuator accessories
- Repair and replace costs
- Added instrumentation
- Education
- Drugs (used in photodynamic therapy)

This isn't a comprehensive list, depending on how the individual facilities develop their departmental cost centers, however; it should aid administration with forecasting the budget for laser use.

Evaluation of the program is objective and subjective. Objectively, we can measure the following; are we meeting the program goals, increasing quality of care, decreasing inpatient days, increasing revenue; education of physician and support staff and utilization of the operating room or outpatient departments. A trends analysis program should be developed, possibly through a case mix management system to document these components. Subjectively, we look at the increasing community awareness of the latest technological advances, at the contribution to clinical research programs and physician education. And at potential increase in publications by physicians, nurses and administrators with regards to the use of lasers in the various treatment modalities, nursing intervention and program effectiveness. Marketing a multi-laser program calls for creative innovation. The use of the media, cable and network television, newspapers, and radio, is usually the most effective technique, however, requires significant cost. Short range marketing approaches include the use of informational brochures, fact sheets, and presentations to community agencies. Another strategy is to develop and implement laser seminars and workshops for physicians, nurses and support personnel. It's important for the continued impetus of a program that the physician community knows and understands the efficacy of laser treatment and equally important is that the community knows how the laser is used in medicine and surgery. This will afford patient a choice of treatment that, ultimately, will be beneficial to them and their families.

The Administrative Role

Administration's commitment to a multi-disciplinary, multi-use laser program must be willing to take financial risks to provide the technology for improved patient care. The medical staff members must be committed to use the lasers in their practice and to take the time it requires to develop, educate and improve the technological delivery of the laser treatment modalities for the delivery of quality patient care.

SUMMARY

Strategic planning and well a designed, developed and implemented feasibility studies must be done before commitment can be made to implement a laser program. Medical Staff commitment is important, and a multi-disciplined laser committee is appointed. The laser committee establishes goals and objectives of the laser program, to include continual monitoring and evaluation of the total scope of laser usage.

Administration continues to work with various departments to develop and cost effective program; including patient charges, reimbursement, procurement of equipment and physician, staff and patient education.

To develop the program's potential, a marketing plan should be developed to increase the awareness of the community of the ultimate benefits of laser treatment modalities. The marketing strategies should include education of physicians, nurses and support personnel to increase the geographical referral scope for the program.

Part 3

Lasers in Medicine and Surgery... The Nurses Role

CHAPTER 8

CLINICAL APPLICATIONS OF LASERS

There are many advantages of laser therapy in surgery and medicine. Some advantages are:

- Pinpoint accuracy when used as a precision tool with the operating microscope.
- Minimal tissue damage.
- Reduced blood loss.
- Reduced infection rate
- Reduced length of stay or done as an outpatient.
- Sealing of the lymphatics
- Cutting or incising tissue with little damage to surrounding tissue.
- Able to coagulate and cut tissue simultaneously.
- Color selectivity.
- Used of the laser through endoscopes to do minimally invasive procedures.
- Use of lasers and a photochemical response to cause tissue necrosis, selectively.

As further research is done, many more advantages for the use of the laser will be developed. As you review the following list of uses for lasers in the various surgical and medical disciplines, understand this isn't an exhaustive compilation of procedures. Many other procedures are being introduced and begun as efficacious on a weekly, even monthly basis.

Generally, lasers either cut, coagulate, vaporize, or ablate tissue. The following is a list of procedures that have clinical applications for the use of the laser.

Dermatology/Plastic Surgery
- Pink hemangiomas
- General hemangiomas
- Capillary/cavernous hemangiomas
- Portwine stains
- Strawberry marks
- Traumatic tattoos excision
- Cutaneous tattoos excision
- Breast surgery
- Augmentation mammoplasty
- Excision of skin lesions

- Excision of benign tumors
- Acne rosacea
- Acne
- Excision of moles and warts
- Spider nevi
- Telangiectasia
- Campbell DeMorgan Senile angiomas
- Pyogenic granuloma
- Burn Eschar
- Debridement of decubitis ulcers

Neurosurgery
- Vascular meningiomas
- Brain tumors, benign or malignant
- Acoustic nerve tumors
- Cerebral gilomas
- Craniopharyngioma
- Spinal cord tumors
- Commissural myelotomy, for intractable pain

Ophthalmology
- Excise scleral tumors
- Dacrocystorhinostomy
- Chalazion excision
- Pterygium excision
- Posterior capsulotomy
- Iridectomies
- Anterior segment strands
- Synechiae
- Photocoagulation of retinal bleeding
- Retinal detachments
- Anterior iridectomies
- Senile macular degeneration
- Retinal tears
- Trabeculoplasty
- Excision of Xanthaloma
- Choreoplasty
- Repair entropion
- Lacrimal punctum
- Pan-endophotocoagulation

Otorhinolaryngology
- Tracheal strictures
- Esophageal webs
- Respiratory papillomatosis
- Juvenile papillomatosis
- Vocal cord nodules
- Polyps vocal cord/nasal
- Vocal cord hyperkeratosis
- Granulomas
- Arytenoidectomy
- Webs and laryngeal stenosis
- Radical neck dissections
- Adult tonsilectomy
- Control of post T & A bleeding
- Tumors of the tongue
- Glossectomy
- Hemilaryngectomy
- Fasioplasty
- Intranasal telangiectasia
- Stapedotomy
- Hemostasis of esophageal bleeding
- Ateriovenous malformation
- Otosclerosis
- Photocoagulation of nasal turbinates
- Choanal atresia

Pulmomary and Thoracic Surgery
- Tumors of the larynx, trachea, and main bronchi
- Lung tumors and wedge resections
- Bronchial Tumors
- Hemorrhagic lesions
- Tracheal stenosis
- Bronchial fistulas
- Destruction of granulomas (chrondomas and adeno mas)
- Decortications
- Coagulation of bleeding lesions
- Ablation of atelectasis or obstructive pneumonities
- Excision of chest wall tumors

Dental and Oral Maxillo-Facial
- Gingivectomy
- Alveoloplasty
- Partial sialodenectomy
- Sialolithotomy
- Excision inta-oral lesion
- Excision sublingual gland
- Laser assisted temporal mandibular arthroplasty
- Ablation of soft tissue lesion, leukoplakia

Gastroenterology
- G.I. Bleeding
- Upper and lower tract tumor ablation
- Recanulization of advanced obstructive tumors
- Esophageal ulcers
- Dudenal ulcer
- Gastric carcinomas
- Gastrointestinal angiomata
- Upper and lower tract polyps
- Gastric erosions
- G.I. vascular malformations
- Treatment of non-bleeding angiodysplasia
- Bleeding varcies
- Esophagitis
- Erosive duduenitis
- Mallory-Weiss Syndrome
- Hemostasis of colonic lesions

General Surgery
- Parathryoidectomy
- Thyroidectomy
- Excision or destruction of intra-abdominal or retro-peritoneal
- tumors/cysts/endometrosis
- Partial hepetectomy
- Tumor surgery
- Excision of matastases of the liver
- Pancreatic Surgery
- Tumors of the abdominal wall
- Varicose ulcers of extremities
- Partial spleenectomy
- Laser assisted Cholecystectomy
- Laser assisted Herniorrhaphy

Clinical Applications of Lasers

- Pilonidal Cystectomy
- Radical Mastectomy

Colon-Rectal Surgery
- Excision of rectal tumors (obstructing)
- Colonic tumors (low lying carcinoma)
- Low risk colon and rectal tumors
- Hemorrhoidectomy
- Anal fistulas and fissures
- Rectal condyloma

Gynecology
- Endometrosis
- Excision of cervical lesions
- Abdominal cysts and tumors
- Tubalplasty
- Wedge resection of the ovaries
- Microlaser myomectomy
- Preinvasive cancer
- Cancer of the cervix, vagina and vulva
- Condyloma accuminata
- Herpes lesions
- Adhesiolysis
- Salpingotomy
- Palliation of Paget's disease of the vulva
- Endometrial ablation for menorrhagia
- Vaginal adenosis
- Closure of rect-vaginal fistula
- Vaginal warts

Orthopedics
- Carpel tunnel syndrome
- Vaporize methyl-methacrylate for re-do total hops
- Laser assisted soft tissue incision for re-do total hips
- Laser assisted arthroscopic procedures

Podiatry
- Warts all types
- Fungus infections
- Ingrown toenails
- Deep rooted calluses
- Painful scars
- Keloids

- Morton's neuroma
- Plantar verrucae
- Porokeratosis
- Partial matrixotomy
- Moasic warts
- Onychonycotic nails
- Debridement of ulcers

Urology
- Condyloma accuminata of penis and anus
- Intra-urethral condyloma accuminata
- Penile and vaginal warts
- Transurethral ablation of large bladder tumors
- Superficial bladder tumors
- Partial nephrectomy
- Fragmentation of urethral stones
- Excision of urethral tissue
- Bladder hemorrhage
- Urethral polyps
- Surgical procedure for Peyronies' disease
- Vasovasotomy
- Oorchectomy
- Adult circumcision

Vascular
- Laser assisted peripheral angioplasty
- Vascular welding

Future Procedures in all Specialities
- Laser recannualization of Coronary Vessels
- Radial Keratotomy
- Fragmentation of biliary calculi
- Photoradiation with bio-chemical dyes for tumor destruction
- Biostimulation to increase wound healing

Not identified in this list is the type of laser used for each procedure. As the research continues we may see more specific wavelengths introduced to do the procedures so it's difficult to predict the laser types. The lasers currently used in medicine and surgery have described in earlier chapters. There will be further discussion on the specific types of laser used in the chapter on perioperative nursing. With the pace that laser technology is being introduced into the medical field, the use of the laser is only limited by the user's mind.

SUMMARY

Lasers are used in almost every medical and surgical discipline. Lasers have a distinct advantage over conventional surgical procedures delivering quality care and giving the physician and patient a choice in treatment modalities. The future for health care is brighten when we can use technological advances to offer patients better medicine and less surgical trauma, by converting many procedures to minimally invasive procedures with the use of laser systems.

CHAPTER 9
THE LASER TEAM

As lasers proliferate in the operating room, the responsibility for their maintenance, safety and effective operation will be assumed by the nursing staff. The multi-use of the laser will call for the assignment of knowledgeable staff members being responsible for the laser. The laser is highly technical equipment and needs special knowledge and skills for maintenance and use without excessive down-time.

Each health care facility will have to assess their ability to appoint specific persons being responsible for the laser. During the needs assessment phase, proposed practical plans should be developed to include; the effect on the surgical schedule, laser utilization, conflict of equipment, and staffing. If the premise of supplying equipment for the physicians to treat patients most appropriately, then all or most of the staff in the laser treatment area should be trained. However, this may be an unrealistic approach, and it's recommended that a preceptor program be developed for the training of staff that may be assigned to assist during laser procedures. The nursing preceptor would be responsible for the training of chosen staff and continued orientation for other personnel that may be involved in the day to day operation of the surgery schedule. The persons title has little relevancy to the position, but several are being used such as; Clinical Laser Nurse, Laser Program Coordinator or Director, Laser Team Leader, or Assistant Head Nurse for Lasers.

As the policies and procedures are established and approved, a laser safety officer should be appointed. This person may be a physician, biomedical technician, the hospital's current radiation safety officer, or the nurse. A team concept can be developed as laser usage increases.

A laser team includes the program leader, biomedical technician, nurses and operating technicians, or other identified persons that can be trained as laser operators in the areas where lasers will be used. The team would receive extensive training and education in aspects of laser technology, applications, safety and their individual responsibilities during a procedure.

To develop the proper job description for each team member, a job analysis should be done. The analysis should include educational requirements, scope and responsibility of each job; experience or skills needed, physical demands, work environment and accountability. A criteria based job description can be developed. The personnel department will be able to review the analysis and factor each position into its proper job and grade for salary designation.

The Laser Team

The *biomedical* or *biolaser* technician job description would include the following:

- Technical training, either in the laser field or in the technical support schools prepared by the manufacturers, or in college or university's that have specific electro-optic programs.
- The ability to do preventive maintenance on the lasers and related equipment.
- Understanding of laser application related to surgical procedures and able to work in a surgical enviroment.
- Good physical health, with good work ethics, with good communication skills.
- Able to comprehend the importance of electrical and non-ionizing radiation safety.
- Has some administrative skills to assume the responsibility for the safety of physicians, patients and support personnel.

The biomedical laser technician can be appointed as the laser safety officer but can also be responsible for laser maintenance and act as a laser operator during the procedure. Other skills would be to understand aseptic techniques, acquire the use of medical terminology and be oriented to the general surgical environment. The biolaser technician would be responsible for participating in the continued education of the nursing and support staff. If the facility has a research program, the biolaser technician would actively participate in the research and/ or development of laser related scientific instruments or delivery systems. Depending of this person's departmental responsibility, he/ she would be responsible to the director of the biomedical department, or the operating room supervisor, or the laser program coordinator.

Another laser team member can be a *laser technician*. The choice of this person could be from the existing staff. An operating room technician usually has applicable skills to work with technical equipment. Further, training related to the knowledge and applications of lasers in medicine and surgery, is minimal. The job description for the laser technician would include such factors as:

- A high school or equivalent education.
- Operating Room Technician skills and related experience.

- Knowledge of laser systems and related instrumentation.
- In good physical health, with good work ethics and communication skills.
- Able to move heavy equipment and understand electrical safety.
- Able to accept responsibility.
- Have good written communication skills to accurately complete documents.
- Have knowledge of the surgical environment understanding the scrub and circulating duties.
- Would help in the continuing education of the physicians, nurses and support staff.

With current experience and knowledge of aseptic technique, the laser technician is a flexible staff member. She/he can be assigned total responsibility for the use of the laser during each procedure. The technician can be used to staff other intra-operative surgical procedures when there are no laser cases on the schedule. The laser technician can also assume the responsibility of the laser safety officer. The laser technician will work with the biomedical or service technician to do preventive maintenance for safe use of the laser and other duties assigned by the clinical laser nurse or program director. Having a registered professional nurse on the laser team compliments effective patient care as she does her/his peri-operative role. This role will be fully described regarding scope and responsibility in the next chapter.

The above job descriptions are intended to describe the general nature and level of work being done. These descriptions aren't considered exhaustive list of all duties did by the personnel in these classifications. Each facility must take a realistic look at their staffing needs and assigned persons qualified to perform the duties of the laser safety officer and or technician.

It's important to consider the education of those persons participating as the laser team. There are formal programs available and several laser manufacturers have developed educational components offered to their costumers as part of the purchase package.

A well organized educational program should "provide didactic and clinical experience for the support staff who will be responsible for the laser during each operative procedure."

The Laser Team

There should be enough time during the program to learn basic, theory of the fundamentals of laser physics and laser application of the various wavelengths to each surgical procedure, and understand the operational characteristics of the laser systems. The education elements for a well structured training program should include:

- Basic laser biophysics.
- Types of laser systems and their tissue effects.
- Advantages of laser surgery in each surgical discipline.
- Laser safety.
- Technical operation or characteristics of lasers. with hands-on experience with each system.
- Trouble shooting techniques.
- Role definition of each team member and an understanding of their responsibilities.
- Administrative responsibilities.

Continuing education for the support staff and team is another component for safe practiced and increased utilization of lasers in medicine and surgery. There are several laser societies being formed in many medical and surgical specialities and laser industry. These societies offer many opportunities for early education as well and continuing education and speciality training course information and are a reliable resource for laser information, generally.

SUMMARY

Lasers are a complex technology that calls for support personnel knowledgeable in their use and maintenance. It's important to identify special persons who will be responsible for the care of the laser and laser safety. The support staff could include a biomedical technician, a laser technician, and an or several registered nurses, anyone could be appointed the Laser Safety Officer. The personnel chosen to maintain the lasers should have specific training in laser technology, electro-optics and the applications of lasers in medicine and surgery.

Although technical schools are available, many manufacturers have their own technical support schools specific for their laser system and offer education opportunities for nurses and physicians. Several laser societies have programs available for the certification and education of physicians. Continued education of physicians, nurses and support staff is paramount for safe practice and increased utilization of the lasers.

CHAPTER 10

THE PERIOPERATIVE LASER NURSE

In 1976, the AORN (Association of Operating Room Nurses) Board of Directors appointed a task force to define the role of the operating room nurse, to make recommendations for operationalization of this role, and to aid in the implementation of the role. The task force presented this definition to the House of Delegates at the 25th AORN Congress and it was approved and adopted.

The following definition is the statement of the perioperative role:

> *"The perioperative role of the operating room nurse consists of nursing activities performed by the professional operating room nurse during the preoperative, intraoperative and post operative phases of the patient's surgical experience. Operating Room nurses assume their perioperative role at a beginning level dependent on their experience and competency to practice As they gain knowledge and skills, they progress on a continuum to an advanced level of practice."* [1]

With the expanded responsibilities in this expanding era of technology, identifying basic competency is essential to providing an understanding of the basic knowledge and skills necessary to fulfill The role of a clinical laser nurse. Defined competency statement provides a base line where the practitioner can progress along a continuum to an expanded role in our nursing practice.

The activities of this role cover three phases; perioperative, intraoperative and post operative. The **preoperative** phase includes an assessment of the patient before he/she is transferred to the surgical environment. Assessment begins in the clinic or office, in the patient's room after admission, by telephone it the patient will be an outpatient or in the holding room in the surgical suite. The **intraoperative** scope of activities include planning with the team to provide necessary instruments, supplies; equipment, positioning requirements and other intraoperative needs for quality care of the patient's surgical intervention. The **post operative** scope of this role is to accompany the patient to the Recovery Room or area of discharge, and give a full report to the person assuming continuing responsibility for the patient, whether the recovery room nurse, ambulatory surgery nurse or the family. A follow-up evaluation, either in the hospital, home or clinic, is important to assess the patient's progress toward wellness.

---

[1] AORN Standards and Recommended Practice for Preoperative Nursing Update. Spring 1983, The Association of Operating Room Nurses, Inc.

Since 1983, when the **American Society for Lasers Medicine and Surgery,** provided for a Nursing Section, they've been working on proposed standards for nursing care for patients having laser procedures. Using basic competency statements the nursing section has proposed nursing standards (yet to be approved by the Board). Basic competency statements have knowledge, skills, and abilities necessary to fulfill, at a minimum level the role of the laser nurse. These standards have been written in broad terms as each practice setting is diverse; patient population varies, as does the environment; services provided and accessibility of resources would influence the criteria and the time for achievement.

The *"laser nurse"* is another nursing specialist, with knowledge and understanding of the technological modality and its use in medicine and surgery. Because nursing is an independent, autonomous, self regulating profession, the primary function of the nurse is to aid sick people to regain health through selective application of nursing knowledge in providing a continuum of competent patient care. The clinical nurse applies this philosophy to patient needing laser surgical interventions. The clinical nurse does her preoperative assessment to include:

- Determining the patient's and the family's knowl edge of the use of lasers for the surgical procedure.
- Assessing the medical history to determine any special equipment or positioning needs during the operation.
- Explaining the various phases of the perioperative plan, including:
  - preoperative medication and expected effects
  - transportation to the Operating Room
  - the wait in the holding room
  - the family's responsibility; what time to arrive, where to wait, etc.
  - the surgical environment
  - what to expect in Recovery Room, i.e., blood pressure every 15 minutes, and the wake up process
- Teaching the patient deep breathing and leg exercises, or specific post operative care depending onthe procedureand what the expected out comes shouldbe.
- Providing psychological support for the patient and family.

The Perioperative Laser Nurse

- Implementing a plan of post operative care for each patient.
- Help in discharge planning.

The intraoperative phase of the nurses' practice includes the implementation of the plan of care and nursing management of the patient during the surgical procedure. It's difficult for the nurse to assume responsibility for circulating duties and laser operation, although during minor procedures, with organization; it is possible. During extensive surgical procedures where the laser is used intermittently, there should be a laser operator as the laser and related equipment calls for the full attention of the support staff who has had the specialized training in all aspects of the laser system. Maintenance of laser safety is paramount during each procedure to provide physical safety for the patient, physician and nursing staff. The clinical nurse assures an aseptically controlled environment, effectively manages other human resources needed during the procedure, positioning of the patient and assures all safety policies and procedures are followed. She also has accountability to assure all equipment, accessories, supplies is readily available for each laser procedure.

The clinical nurse, laser technician or biomedical technician is responsible for the operation of the laser during each procedure. This responsibility includes a pre-use check out procedure, assuring the laser is functional before each uses. Should the laser not be functioning, the operating room supervisor is notified immediately, so the physician can be notified and an adjustment in the schedule made for continued expedition of the operative schedule. The laser check out list includes:

- Laser available.
- Electrical power to system.
- Laser gas level checked, tank changes if necessary.
  (this depends of the type of laser system)
- Check the spot size and co-axial aiming beam.
- Assure the handpieces are sterile.
- Have smoke evacuator available with necessary attachments.
- Have the proper instrumentation and accessories to do the procedures.
- Check the micromanipulator and objective lenses.
- Position the laser for the procedure.

Documentation of the laser use during each case is important as a medical/legal responsibility, but also, for accumulative clinical information. A laser log, or nursing documentation on the proper form is kept for each laser and this information should include:

- name and I.D. number
- physician and any assistants
- type of anesthesia
- note if special laser shield endotracheal tube was used
- all safety rules adhered to, such as glasses on, signs on doors, viewing windows covered
- type of procedure being done
- type of laser used
- all energy settings noted, changes documented
- total time laser was used
- signature of laser operator

A section for comments should be included for further documentation of events that may have happened during the case.

The clinical nurse offers psychological support for the patient during the intraoperative phase, especially if the patient is awake during the laser treatment. Another responsibility of the laser operator during the procedure, is to put the laser in a stand-by mode when the physician isn't using the laser. The stand-by mode is safe practice as the physician can't accidently fire the laser as this mode "disables" the operation of the beam exit.

The continued responsibility of the clinical nurse is to accompany the patient to the Recovery Room. She gives the recovery room nurse a full report of the laser procedure that was done during the operation. If the patient is an outpatient, the clinical nurse accompanies the patient to the outpatient department and gives a full report to the nurses and the patient's family. The circulating nurse assumes her normal intraoperative responsibilities, if not the laser operator, during the laser procedure.

The post operative phase of the perioperative role is the evaluation of the patient's response to the surgical intervention. If the patient is in the hospital post operatively, they're visited by the nurse to assess the patient's satisfaction and progress to wellness. As an outpatient, a telephone assessment is necessary. The clinical nurse worked with the outpatient or clinic nurses to develop discharge instructions for the patient and family. (see appendix) The clinical nurse is the link from the patient and his/her family to the physician, for continued support

The Perioperative Laser Nurse

in the patient's return to the activities of daily living. Patient assessment is a continuous activity to identify the patient's needs or problems and to help the physician in the efficient and effective perioperative care. In this, the clinical nurse's role is invaluable. The nursing process provides us with a systematic approach of safe nursing practice and quality care is the result.

The clinical nurse assumes many other duties in relation to laser surgery. She/he has the responsibility of the daily supervision of the para-professional team. This may include scheduling their time for the most efficient assignments for each laser procedure. She/he also supervises the cleaning and maintenance of laser related accessories, instruments, and equipment. The clinical nurse assures the laser shut down procedure is complete and the laser is store appropriately. She/he also executes the performance evaluation of the team, sits on the Laser Committee, participates in the quality assurance process and can be involved in research projects on laser procedures. If the facility is participating in investigational protocols and needs completion of various reports that must be sent to the F.D.A., the nurse verifies all the documentation is complete and submitted to the proper authorities or available for review when requested.

The clinical nurse participates in on going educational programs for physicians, nurses and support staff. She/he aids in the development of patient information handbooks and home instructions for discharge planning. The nurse has the responsibility for the development, implementing and up-dating of laser related policies and procedures. The clinical nurse can be involved in physician marketing assuring increased awareness and usage of the various laser wavelengths. The scope of her position is far reaching and is a resource for her colleagues in planning the care of patients having laser therapy during their surgical intervention.

SUMMARY

The role of the operating room nurse having been defined as the "perioperative role" by their professional organization gives the operating room nurse direction in his/her practice. There are three phases described in the role definition; preoperative, intraoperative and post operative. Using the nursing process of assessment, planning implementation and evaluation the clinical nurse is a specialist in her practice. She provides the patient link to the physician as she/he assesses the patient's psychological needs, reviews the medical history to develop and intraoperative plan of care, executes the plan during the surgical intervention and evaluates the patient's progress to wellness. As a specialist, she/he participates in the supervision of the laser team, develops, implements and updates policies and procedures, in continuing education programs and in the development of patient education information and is a valuable member of the Laser Committee. As the laser specialist she/he is also responsible for the education of her nursing colleagues, as they need information about the affect of the laser on patient care. The continued education and orientation of the nursing staff in the various departments where laser procedures are done is also the clinical nurse's responsibility. The clinical nurse is unique to her speciality and shares her practice knowledge with her colleagues.

CHAPTER 11

PRE, INTRA, AND POST OPERATIVE CARE OF PATIENTS ... HAVING LASER PROCEDURES

The nursing aspect of laser surgery is divided into three distinct sections; preoperative, intraoperative and post operative, each using a defined phase of the nursing process. The nursing process incorporates four segments of care; assessment, planning, implementation and evaluation. The patient having surgery, to include the use of lasers, are prepared with care that incorporates the nursing process.

SECTION I

Nursing Assessment

Preoperative care for patients needing the use of the laser in their surgical intervention isn't essentially different for patients having conventional surgical procedures.

Preoperative assessment of the patient's understanding of the use of the laser during his/her operative procedure is of paramount importance. Giving the patient and family the opportunity to verbalize their fears and anxieties and responding appropriately to this behavior is an important role of the clinical nurse. The advantages of laser surgery was discussed in Chapter 8, of this book.

Preoperative teaching is an opportunity for the nurse to reinforce the physician's explanation of the surgical procedure and assess the patient's understanding of his/her hospitalization and surgical intervention. The nurse must take time with the patient or family and listen to them, avoiding medical jargon and standard cliches while explaining the expected risks and outcomes of the procedure, or teaching them techniques for deep breathing, turning, incisional support, leg exercises and how to ambulate can be demonstrated and the patient's comprehension can be assessed by having them return the demonstration. Explanation of the progressive care will encourage early ambulation and self care. This will be the opportunity to begin developing the discharge plan and confirm the patient or family member understands the post surgical care and its implication to daily activities. Discuss with the patient and family the regulations of the hospital, visiting hours, numbers of visitors, location of waiting rooms, where the visitors bathrooms are located and the cafeteria hours or the vending locations through out the hospital. The family should understand the approximate lengths of time the patient will be away from the nursing unit, and the approximate lengths of time in the holding room for the operative procedure and that the Recovery Room should notify them when the patient comes. Explain to the family where to wait and how the physician will contact them when the operation is finished. The patient needs to understand pain management, so an explanation of the medication ordered and how it may affect him/her, is important. Make sure to note the patient's religious preference and ask if they wish to see the chaplain or have their own minister, priest or rabbi notified.

Preoperative care will include preparing the patient for the surgical procedure, usually with an antibacterial bath or shower; maybe ordering an enema or bowel prep, taking and recording vital signs, checking and noting allergies, completing proper lab work with reports on the chart, completing X-rays and electrocardiograms, as ordered, completed history and physical, and ordering blood, if needed. The patient should be NPO after midnight or as ordered and an informed consent should be signed, witnessed and on the chart. Before the patient is transported to surgery, have the patient urinate, remove dentures, contact lens, prothesis, nail polish and make-up, and assure all valuables are secured.

After the preoperative medication is given, pull up the side rails, turn off the light or pull the blinds so the patient can rest in a subdued, quiet atmosphere. Complete the chart, including the patients addressograph plate and remind the patient's family where to wait while the patient is in the operating room.

The ambulatory surgery preoperative procedure differs in scope. Usually, the preoperative preparation is done before of the admission. Nursing assessment is done either in a pre-admission interview and seen by the anesthesiologist, also, or a telephone assessment is done. Ambulatory patients are either given instructions at the physician's office or sent pre-admission instructions. These instructions would include; where the entrance to the out patient department is located and where to proceed from there; time of arrival, what **not to** bring to the hospital and being assured the patient was accompanied by a responsible person to escort them home. The brochure or telephone instructions give explanations of the risks and expected outcomes of the surgical procedure and usually included, using the laser for the surgical intervention.

The Perioperative Care of Patients

When the patients are scheduled for admissions the laser should be listed including any other special equipment, to avoid conflict of use. It would also be useful to include other pertinent equipment that might be needed during the case, approximate time the laser would be used to plan for continued usage throughout the daily schedule. The physician laser privilege list should be kept in or near the scheduling book and updated as needed.

Surgical Preoperative Assessment

As the patient comes in the holding area of the operating room, continued preoperative care is given. The chart is checked for completeness and any deficiencies are corrected before the patient being transferred to the operating room table.

In the holding area, the anesthesiologist re-assesses the patient, starts parenteral fluids, inserts other intravenous lines proper, the shave prep can be done, as needed and the circulating nurses introduces her/him self to the patient and makes proper verification of the patient's identity and identification of the surgical procedure being done. The patient is transferred to the operating room table with the circulating nurse in attendance always. She/he assures the patient's right to privacy, safety and comfort, staying with the patient always and helping the anesthesiologist during induction and intubation of the patient.

Outpatient Assessment

The outpatient has minimal preoperative preparation and instructional opportunities before his/her surgical intervention. Most ambulatory surgery patient receive instructions via the physician's office or clinic nurse. Most outpatient centers, either self contained or integrated units have waiting area for the patient's family and a physician consultation room for post operative family contact. The ambulatory surgery patient receives post-operative discharge home instructions (see appendix), by the nurse in the outpatient department. Follow-up post-operative evaluation of the outpatient can be done by telephone either by the clinical nurse or the outpatient nurse liaison. A patient survey can be given to the patient, being returned by mail, assessing the care given while in the hospital milieu.

Post-operative care for the inpatient begins as he/she comes in the Post-Anesthesia (Surgical) Recovery Room. The clinical nurse or the circulating nurse gives a full report to the nursing staff in the Recovery Room. The patient is transferred to their nursing unit after meeting certain post anesthesia criteria.

SECTION II

Intraoperative Responsibilities

Developing and implementing the intraoperative care plan takes knowledge and understanding of each surgical procedure and the treatment application of the laser.

The tremendous advancements in the care of the surgical patient, the sophistication of anesthesiology, understanding of the causes and effect of infections, advances in the pharmacotherapeutics, new diagnostic techniques, and the implementation of high technology in surgical specialties have resulted in safe, exacting and professional skills being applied in the treatment of patients needing surgical interventions.

The maintenance of the aseptic surgical environment is the prime role of the operating room nurse. The implementation of the care plan for each surgical intervention assures that each patient will receive individualized, competent care.

The intraoperative care of the patient having laser surgery is directly related to his/her surgical procedure (further operative information will be described in Section III). Each physicians surgical set up has preference cards and the laser is used as adjunctive equipment to specific procedures.

The patient is positioned and his/her skin is prepped according to the physician's preference. Care of each patient during the positioning should include avoidance of unnecessary exposure and loss of dignity, and adequate exposure of the operative site. The anesthesiologist must be able to maintain a patent airway and have optimum ventilation.

The patient must have protection from nerve and muscle pressure, maintenance of circulation to all area, prevention of unnecessary chilling and proper placement of the electro-cautery grounding plate. When scrubbing the operative site, make sure to note that the patient isn't allergic to any of the bacteriostatic agents being used. Proper scrubbing of the operative site assures a bacteria free operative area, scrubbing from the proposed incision site to the periphery of the field.

The laser may not be routinely used as an incisive tool, and doesn't need to be moved into the field until such a time as it'll be used. The clinical nurse or laser safety officer's responsibility is to have the laser in surgical readiness. The following steps should be taken before the operative procedure:

Immediately, Before the Procedure
- Laser available for procedure and pre-operative check done
- Handpiece attached or
- Laser connected to the microscope
- Laser draped as necessary
- Smoke evacuator tubing, wand, or filter on cart
- Signs in place on all entrances to suite
- Viewing windows covered, as necessary
- Eye protection available for staff of correct optical density

The Procedure
- Check out procedure finished
- Laser in room immediately accessible
- Microscope checked, working, set-up, with proper objective lens
- Smoke evacuator in room, set up ready to be used
- Clinical Nurse, laser technician or laser safety officer inroom or as laser operative and defined by policy

On Procedure Card
- Handpiece sterilized
- Endoscopes available, checked and in working order
- Fibers soaking and sterile if needed
- Fibers, handpieces and probes identifie per procedure
- Drapes for laser or microscope
- Any other special instruments identified and avail able

Post Operatively
- Laser shut off
- Accessories disassembled and cleaned according to procedures
- Accessories wiped off and appropriately stored
- Smoke evacuator cleaned and supplies restocked
- Documentation done

As each laser and laser procedures may need different accessories and equipment being used during the operative procedure, the above list isn't all inclusive. Other laser information can be added to the physician's preference card as he/she uses the laser for various procedures in their surgical practice. Pictures or detailed descriptions of room and laser set up can be attached to the procedure cards that may aid in continuity for expediting the procedure.

Medications may be prescribed and should be available for laser procedures. Some of these medications are: 37% acetic acid, dilute solution of vasopressin, toluidine blue, Lugol's solution, hyskon, and local anaesthetics, as ordered.

Outpatient may need some same procedural set-ups and instrumentation. Typically, the outpatient will have to be monitored during the procedure, automatic blood pressure equipment is efficient and give the circulating nurse more freedom to do her/his duties.

The CO_2 laser has minimal instrumentation and accessory requirements for each case. Water stops the CO_2 laser beam and protects surrounding tissue, so extra irrigation solution should be available. Also, towels or laparotomy pads should be soaked in irrigation solution and packed around the incision site and surrounding tissue. When using the CO_2 laser around the rectum, it's recommended a saline soaked gauze pack or tampon be put into the rectum to prevent methylene gas explosion. The quartz or titanium rods are used to manipulate tissue or as back-stops for the CO_2 laser beam, when vaporizating tissue. If the tissue "sticks" to the rod, a little irrigation fluid will float it free. Quartz or titanium rods are preferred as they absorb the laser energy on impact and won't break. Glass rods are avoided as the laser energy can shatter them. When the quartz rods have multiple impact marks, they should be discarded, as they can break from energy fatigue.

Vaporization of tissue with the CO_2 and Nd: YAG laser causes smoke or "plume," and a smoke evacuation system should be available always. The tubing is sterile and passed onto the operative field. If only a small area is being vaporized, the hospital vacuum system may be used. However, to preserve the integrity of the vacuum system, a filter should be placed between the canister and the vacuum manifold. These plume filters are available in large and small sizes. The filter should be changed after each day unless and excessive number of laser procedures are in that operating room, in which case the filter should be changed more frequently. All filters and disposable items used during a laser procedure when patient has HIV, condyloma, herpes or other highly transmittable diseases, contaminated case

The Perioperative Care of Patients

techniques are used and all disposable equipment treated by established bio-hazard procedures.

The Nd: YAG laser has a complement of accessories that can be used separately or with a variety of endoscopes. The endoscopes used with the laser are any fiberscopes readily available on the market. The laser fiber is passed down the biopsy channel, assuring the fiber tip is well beyond the end of the scope. If the fiber isn't extended beyond the tip of the fiberscope, the fiber and/or the scope tip can be burned. It's recommended that all fiberscopes be fitted with a laser-protected tip to prevent absorption of the energy generated by the laser fiber. The bare fiber tip may burn or be destroyed if inserted into the tissue. The fiber will have to be changed and the tip cut and polished before it can be reused. Most manufacturers of the fibers have cutting and polishing kits available and the laser technician or biomedical personnel are taught to cut and polish fibers. The other choice for repair of the fibers is to return them to the manufacturer for repair that's costly. The fibers, whether used as contact or non-contact, are washed with warm soapy water, inspected for integrity and can be sterilized in ethylene oxide or soaked in Cidex tm. There are several pre-packaged sterile disposable fibers available. The contact laser tips must be inspected for integrity, as they lose energy transmission if broken or burned. The endoscopes are cleaned and reprocessed between patients by the manufacturer's recommendations and the hospitals decontamination, cleaning and sterilization procedure.

The Argon Laser for Dermato-Plastic Surgery has a collimated hand piece that's soaked in Cidex[tm] before using. After patient uses, it's washed in warm soapy water and re-soaked in the bacteriocidal solution or can be terminally sterilized by ethylene oxide.

The ophthalmology laser needs little attention, except the general external cleaning each day. The gonioscopic lenses used with the eye laser are cleaned carefully with absolute alcohol and lens paper before patient uses, also, examined for pitting, as any defect may deflect the laser beam.

Instrumentation for each laser procedure is specific for that surgical intervention. It's recommended that instruments used for laser surgery is anodized or matte finished to reduce inappropriate laser beam deflection. Many instrument and laser companies have these instruments readily available, however; many companies will cooperate with the facility and refinish picked instruments, as needed.

Standard instrument set-ups are usually determined by physician preference. There are a few special instruments specific and may be new to each specialty some of these instruments are:

- Suspension systems for oropharynx/larynx procedures
- Miniaturized forceps, cups and probes with 22cm handles
- Foot plates as back stops
- Special eye protection
- Special laser shielded endotracheal tubes
- Micromanipulators with a variety of objective lens
- Laser bronchoscopes
- Laser laparoscopes with additional puncture trocars
- Flexible endoscopes with 2.6 mm channels
- Smoke evacuator equipment
- Vaginal speculum, anodized/matte finished
- Angled and straight long calipers
- Albarran's Bridge as a fiber guide used in Gyne and Urology
- Quartz or Titanium rods with various angles
- Silver sided dental or rhodium mirrors
- Gonioscopic lens for ophthalmology

The above list isn't exhaustive for laser surgery, as new procedures are developed the need for other instrumentation and accessories will have rapid growth.

The technical responsibility of the clinical nurse during surgical intervention is to maintain the integrity of the surgical field, to provide help, as needed to the anesthesiologist, surgeon and scrub nurse, to document the nursing events that happen during the procedure, including the laser related activity, intake and output of fluids, medications administered and to take sponge, needle and instrument counts. The nursing responsibilities will continue to assess, monitor and evaluate on activities of the patient care plan and adjust in the plan as the surgical intervention proceeds, to maintain patient safety and assure quality patient care.

The circulating nurse may have the additional responsibility of being the laser operator. This adds other tasks during the intraoperative care of the patient. A recommendation to enhance expediting the laser procedure, is that the facility assess the staffing patient and acuity of the case and adjust for more staffing during a laser procedure, as needed. Depending, on laser usage other staff members will have to become laser trained to accommodate safe operation of the laser systems. Laser trained personnel have the responsibility for safe practice during each procedure. Some facilities have designated laser operators who gives their full attention to laser operation during the procedure and when there are no laser cases scheduled assigned other duties, this provides more flexibility to normal staffing patterns. The circulating nurse continues to have responsibility of discharging the patient from the operating room and helps in removing the drapes, grounding pads, restraints and positioning supplies. The patient should be washed-up, a clean gown and covered with a warm blanket, keeping the patients body in good alignment while transferring the patient to the post-anesthesia bed. Documentation of the procedure is another responsibility for the professional nurse. Information regarding the use of the laser during the procedure must be noted. A laser log can be developed as a separate document or the laser information added to the nursing notes. (see Laser Log in Appdendix)

The continued responsibility of the clinical nurse is to accompany the patient to the post-anesthesia recovery room (PARR), with a report to the nurse in PARR explaining any nursing implication that may have happened during the procedure, to included any unusual occurrences during the laser treatment.

The most serious complication to happen during laser surgery would be an endotracheal fire, during intraoral or areodigestive procedures. Two types of burn injury are produced by laser explosion; thermal and chemical. The first is related to the flame, second by the carbonaceous debris from the endotracheal tube. If an endotracheal fire happens the following steps should be taken:

- REMOVE THE ENDOTRACHEAL TUBE
- GIVE MUSCLE RELAXENTS
- RE-INTUBATE IMMEDIATELY
- DISCONNECT THE O2 FROM BURNNING TUBE
- EXTINGUISH ANY BURNNING ELEMENTS
- INSPECT RESPIRATORY SYSTEM
- ADMINISTER PROPER DRUGS
- HAVE TRACHEOTOMY TRAY AVAILABLE
- KEEP CALM !!
- DOCUMENT OCCURRENCE

By immediately giving muscle relaxants and re-intubating the patient it's hoped that a laryngospasm may be prevented. If there's extensive airway damage a tracheostomy may be necessary. The damage is done primarily to the larynx, epiglottis and across the base of the tongue. The flame may also burn the lips and face as the burning endotracheal tube is being removed. The lips and face area can be covered by a wet towel or laparotomy sponge that will help prevent extensive damage. Usually, large doses of antibiotics and corticosteroids are administered. A lung scan may be necessary to assess the total injury to the respiratory system.

A policy and procedure, should an endotracheal fire happen, should be developed with a multi-disciplinary approach. It'd be reviewed frequently and all members of the surgical team made aware of their duties. This patient may be admitted to the surgical intensive care unit for further observation.

When laser patients are in the PARR, on going care is given. Level of conciousness is assessed, vital signs taken and recorded, parenteral fluids are checked for infusion rates, integrity of the incision site checked, and all drainage tubes are checked with intake and output recorded. The post operative orders are checked and begun. When the patient has met the discharge from PARR criteria and is seen by the anesthesiologist, they're discharged accordingly, either to their inpatient unit or to the outpatient unit.

The family is notified that the patient is in the PARR by the physician or nurse liaison. When the patient is stable the family may visit if that's policy or is sent to the patient's room or proper waiting area, until the patient is discharged from PARR. If the patient is an inpatient, before his/her discharge from PARR is nurse telephones the unit of give them a status report that includes; level of consciousness, vital signs, fluid intake and output, condition of operative site, any drains and where they're found, and any unusual occurrences either in the operating room or PARR. If the inpatient unit is ready to accept the patient they're transferred to the unit for continued care.

If the patient is an outpatient, they may be discharged for the outpatient department of the facility. Normally, the patient isn't discharged until there's no vomiting, able to walk without assistance, and has had pain management. The discharge instructions are given by the clinical nurse and explained to the patient and a family member. The patient shouldn't be discharged from the facility unless accompanied by a responsible person.

The Perioperative Care of Patients

General discharge instructions are:

- CHECK OPERATIVE SITE FOR DRAINAGE
- DRINK FLUIDS AND EAT LIGHTLY, FIRST DAY
- DON'T OPERATE A VECHICLE FOR 24 HOURS
- DON'T SIGN IMPORTANT DOCUMENTS
- AVOID ALCOHOLIC BEVERAGES
- CALL DOCTOR, FOR UNUSUAL OCCURRENCE
- KEEP SCHEDULED APPOINTMENT

The patient should also be instructed on what the expected outcomes should be for his/her procedures so they'll be able to assess an "unusual occurrence." If they're unable to reach their physician for any reason they'd be instructed to return to the facilities emergency room. Specific discharge instructions can be developed as a patient self-care prescription to take with him/her as a check list to follow when they return home. The follow-up for outpatient's having laser or other procedures can be by telephone, the first and possibly the third post operative day, information about the patients progress to wellness is documented on the patient's medical record.

SECTION III

Specific Laser Procedural Information

Most patients having laser surgery doesn't have special perioperative events. There's much documentation that laser patients have, less pain, although this theory, being subjective, has yet to be confirmed. It's believe there's less trauma to the tissue during the procedure, reducing post operative discomfort, it's difficult to quantify as each patient's level of pain tolerance is different.

To help nursing personnel, having the responsibility of the continuity of patient care, I'll try to identify post operative assessment, evaluation criteria and suggest nursing intervention for patients having laser procedures.

Neurosurgical, there seem to be no systemic or cerebral adverse effects related to patients having laser therapy. Although there's limited use of the laser in neurosurgery, when proper, it's the treatment of choice in most extra-axial tumors, in intra-axial tumors for excision or debulking, aneurism shrinkage, neuro-ablative procedures, soft tissue, vascular anomalies, and more recently in selected ventricular tumor ablation. Vaporizing, or excising cerbral tumors with the laser takes less time and damage to surrounding tissue is minimal. Laser surgical resection has less blood loss, reducing operative time and is associated minimal cerebral edema. Using the CO_2 laser, the procedure for extra-axial tumors is as follows:

ROOM SET UP, ACCOMMODATES ALL EQUIPMENT

STANDARD CRANIOTOMY INSTRUMENT SET UP
- instruments matte or anodized
- cottonoid patties counted (all sizes)
- irrigation solution, special suction, fluid/smoke
- microscope and laser drapes
- micromanipulator/objective lens
- prepped in usual manner, dried before draping patient draped in usual fashion, without plastic drapes

EXPOSURE OF TUMOR THROUGH LIMITED CRANIOSTOMY
- centered over accessible part of neo-plasm

METICULOUS DISSECTION AVOIDING DAMAGE TO VITAL STRUCTURES ALLOWING FOR TUMOR REMOVAL
- laser vaporization/hemostasis/shrinkage
- laser allows devitalization of site attachment

Using the laser avoids damage to vessels, nerves and allows complete removal of the tumor. The tumor is either excised or vaporized and shrinkage of the capsule is obtained by using a defocused mode.

Clinical recovery from laser neurosurgical procedures is usually good, with no further expectation of neurologic abnormalities. The post operative neurosurgical course is usually uneventful which is attributed to the no-touch technique, reduced retraction of tissue and cerebral edema, precise vaporization of tissue and internal decompression of the tumor is minimized with hemostatic control, and many patients have reduce length of stay in the intensive care unit.

Immediate post operative care includes orders to; maintain airway, elevate the head of the bed 30-45 degrees, check vital and neuro signs and report any changes in the vital signs or levels of unconsciousness to the physician, immediately. Parenteral fluids will be maintained and medications administered, usually steroids, anti-convulsants and analgesics, avoiding narcotics. Seizure precautions are maintained, intake and output measured, proper lab studies continued, dressings checked, reinforced or changed, as necessary. Nursing care is to continue with oral suctioning, as needed, turning the patient every two hours or in a special reduced pressure bed, with skin care and

The Perioperative Care of Patients

oral hygiene, given. As the patient awakens, orient them to surroundings and time.

On-going care includes increased activity as ordered and as indicated by the patient's status. Range of motion exercises should be passive or active as indicated, with coughing and deep breathing encouraged. Pain management and progressive diet, are also suggested. The patient usually progresses through convalescent care rapidly and is encouraged to return to activities of daily living shows that his/her progress to wellness.

Patient teaching and discharge criteria ensure that the patient and his/her family know and understand the nature and conditions of the illness, the names and actions of medications, exercise tolerance, the importance of assisting the performance of self-care, how to care for the surgical incision, and how to report concerns to the physician. The patient and family need to know the importance of on-going out patient care.

OPHTHALMOLOGY Ophthalmologists have been the for runners in the application of laser to medicine. Currently, ophthalmologists are using three types of surgical lasers; the Argon-ion, with Krypton as an additional choice, Nd: YAG and a Tunable Dye laser. Procedures done with the Argon and YAG lasers are done on an outpatient basis, often in the physician's office. Nurses working in outpatient surgery or clinics usually have responsibility for the ophthalmology patients.

The patient may or may not have local anesthesia administered before the laser procedure. However, retrobulbar anesthesia of 2% lidocaine may be administered and a gonioscopic lens inserted as the patient sits before a slit lamp, resting their chin on the chin-rest. Laser treatment is applied using photocoagulation or photodisruption for the therapy, depending on the etiology. Patients having Argon laser procedures may have diabetic retinopathy or glaucoma, when the YAG laser is used they may have a secondary cataract and need a posterior capsulotomy. When using the Argon lasers the procedures may take from 20-45 minutes with the patient holding perfectly still, a most uncomfortable position, especially for out gerontological patients.

Patients having laser treatment for glaucomas may have slight localized corneal edema and perilimbal congestion may develop during the treatment. Post operative ice bags applied to the site for twenty minutes may reduce the edema and post laser discomfort. Intraocular pressure is measured at intervals of one to two days during the first post operative week.

With minimal inflammatory response produced by the laser beam, healing of the trabecular meshwork and its endothelium plays and important role in reversing the hypotensive effect in the open-angle glaucoma group.

The Kyrpton laser is usually an adjunct to the Argon laser as an option to produce a monochromatic yellow or red beam to treat ophthalmic vascular and choroidoretinal abnormalities. With the Krypton laser, less energy is needed to produce vascular spasm or coagulation. Subsequently, choroidoretinal vascular lesions can be treated with less regard to the filtering or scattering effect of corneal, lenticular or vitreal opacities or the hazard of excessive absorption of high energy beams, to these structures.

Another Argon laser treatment is for diabetic retinopathy, a serious, visual disability that's the leading cause of blindness, in diabetic patients. This laser treatment is also an outpatient procedure. This is a simple, low-risk treatment that delays visual deterioration in patient with retinal neo-vascularization.

The Nd: YAG laser used either as a mode locked (limited dynamic range) or Q-switched (high energy) laser permits microsurgical incision of the posterior capsule without surgery. It's theorized that 30-50% of all patients having intra-ocular lens procedures will need a posterior capsulotomy.

Immediate care post laser treatment is; to check the patient's vital signs, making use they've had no reaction if a local anaesthetic was administered, possibly apply ice bags to the eye for reduction in intraocular pressure and reduced discomfort. Potential complications may be; bleeding, increased intraocular pressure, retinal problems or "pitting of the lens. Patients may be discharged to a responsible person after discharge instruction has been given.

Discharge instructions are divided into several categories; they may include the following:

MEDICATION	EYE CARE	ACTIVITY
NONE UNLESS ORDERED BY PHYSICIAN	REMOVE PATCH 2nd POST OP DAY	LIMITED FOR 2 POST LASER DAYS
TYENOL Q.I.D. AS NEEDED	APPLY WARM COMPRESSES	AVOID SUN LIGHT
APPLY ICE BAG FOR DISCOMFORT	WEAR SUNGLASSES RESUME DIET	NO LIFTING

The patient should understand his/her treatment, how and when to administer their eye medication, what symptoms are important to not-ify the physician, to avoid rubbing, touching or bumping the eye, and the importance of on-going outpatient care. Immediate post laser ex-pectations may be; blurred vision, after-flash, slight headache, irritation of the eye, see "floaters" and eye sensitivity. There have been no reported complications from the posterior capsulotomy procedure and has been safely done with satisfaction, as most patients believe a "miracle" has happened.

The use of the tunable dye laser in the adjunctive treatment of choroidal melanomas has seemed to be effective. Former treatment of the malignant disease resulted in enucleation. This may be an inpatient procedure, the patient receive an intravenous injection of hematoporphyrin derivative, (HpD) about 36-48 hours before their laser treatment.

The HpD leeches out of normal cells, but is selectively absorbed in tumor cells. The tunable dye laser, at 633 nm, is delivered to the eye through a quartz fiber, with or with out a cylindrical diffuser, for about 40 minutes. The laser beam causes a biochemical response to the HpD, causing singlet oxygen to occur within the tumor cells, causing tumor necrosis. Immediate post operative reaction is; peri-orbital edema, as the laser beam creates minimal thermal response. The dye that's injected causes photosensitivity and the patient must stay out of the direct sunlight for about 30-45 days. The patient should be encouraged to use sun screen lotions on exposed areas and to wear long sleeves; pants and a hat should they go out side. They'd be instructed to do their outside activities in the evening, whenever possible, during the time. Then return slowly to their out side activities continuing to use sun screen lotions.

Otolaryngology There are distinct advantages for patients having intra-oral laser surgery. Surgical precision offered with the microscope and lack of bleeding allows maximum excision of the lesion with the preservation of normal tissue. There are uses in otolaryngology for several types of lasers. The specialty of otorhinolaryngology, includes ears, nose, throat, oral cavity; to include the larynx, pharynx, trachea, the neck and the skin of the external structures. Subsequently, physicians in this specialty often sub-specialize.

The Argon laser, producing visible light in the blue-green wave lengths, are strongly absorbed by hemoglobin and pigmented tissue. The Argon laser produces a blanching of the vascular lesions, causing coagulation of the vascular bed in Port Wine Stains, Hemangiomas, Telangiectasia and epistaxis.

The Otologist focuses the Argon laser beam to a small spot size to do Stapedotomy procedures, because of its ability to focus into a very small beam other middle ear procedures can be done, such as; lysis of adhesions, ossicle sculpturing and spot welding of tympanic grafts.

The Nd: YAG laser in the near infrared, with its ability being transmitted through clear liquids ar material, and with the use of the sapphire ceramic contact probes, tissue in the oral cavity, trachea, larynx, pharynx and large tissue masses can be excised, vaporized or coagulated. The convenience of using the YAG wavelength is that it can also be transmitted through flexible quartz fibers and pass down rigid or flexible endoscopes, managing upper airway obstructing lesions difficult to reach or may have a bleeding diaphasis.

The Carbon Dioxide laser has been used since 1972 in otolaryngology and was the first to precisely vaporize vocal cord lesions. Patients having surgical procedures where the CO_2 laser is used are usually anthestized so they hold perfectly still and the laser beam is transmitted via rigid endoscopes such as laryngoscopes or bronchoscopes. The laser is connected directly through the endoscopes or to the microscope by the micromanipulator. At the present time, there's limited use of the CO_2 laser transmitted via a flexible fiber optic.

Subsequently, the speciality of Otolaryngology has a choice of wavelengths for a variety of procedures.

The intraoperative responsibilities for otolaryngology procedures are multiple, as the operating room equipment must be placed for convenience and good visualization of the intra oral lesions. The operating room table must be stabilized and an emergency cart with a tracheostomy tray available should an endotracheal fire happen. The protocol to handle an endotracheal tube explosion has been discussed in the earlier chapter on Laser Safety. Several companies have tried to address the production of anti-flammable tubes, however the best approach is a team effort, understanding each laser wavelength and that safety guidelines have been established and are approved protocols.

For **Subglottic Procedures,** the following is a list of supplies and equipment that may be used during these procedures:

EQUIPMENT	INSTRUMENTS	SUPPLIES
CO_2 Laser	Microlaryngeal Laryngoscope (s)	Cottonoids
Smoke Evacuator	Operating Platform	10F RedRubber Catheter

The Perioperative Care of Patients

CPR Cart	Cord Roller
Laser Protected Endo Tube	Subglottic Mirrors
	Grasping Forceps
	Cup Forceps
	Probes Straight/Angles

Using a red rubber catheter with more openings along the side, attached to the smoke evacuation system is small enough being in the oral cavity and helps in efficient smoke evacuation.

Post operatively, there's a slight inflammatory response, little or no postoperative pain and undelayed healing. The operative time is reduced and major resections of tissue can be done without skin incisions or the need for tracheostomy. The laser plume can be evacuated through the suction channel of the laryngoscope in the oral cavity. Intra-oral operative sites heal within one week and epithelialization is complete after three weeks. It's theorized that rapid healing and epithelialization are resulting from minimal disturbance of adjacent tissue. This also results in decreased post operative scarring. Patients having laser procedures on their larynx have noticed their hoarseness uniformally improved on the first postoperative day. Patients who has other intra-oral laser procedures for cancer, papillomas, and vocal cord polyps are usually discharged on their first or second post operative day with normal alimentation, useful voices and needing no analgesics. Patients having their vocal cord polyps removed usually have their voices promptly restored to their normal speaking voice before surgery.

However, the patient should stick to the program of voice rest for one week, gradual resumption of voice use for the next two weeks, and a complete avoidance of whispering, singing, yelling or talking when there's a high noise level. This presents a major task for patients and frequently calls for absence from work, but the regime will be beneficial for the patients.

Choanalatresia is a defect that's partial or complete persistence of the buccopharyngeal membrane, causing nasal obstruction. It's associated with newborn morbidity. Transnasal resection of the membrane with the CO_2 laser has become the treatment of choice. A saline-soaked cottonoid is placed in the nasopharynx and the atresia is vaporized until the neurosurgical sponge is visualized in the oropharynx. A polyvinyl stent may have to be placed. The stent is maintained from two to six weeks; the nasal passages must be cleaned and suctioned at regular intervals. The patient should have adequate humidification supplied during this time to prevent crusting.

Other areas of treatment in **Otolaryngology** include:

Tracheal Stenosis for scar and soft tissue removal, the laser is efficient resulting from excellent hemostasis. However, recurrent scarring remains a problem. Usually, supplemental treatment must be included, such as; periodic dilation, use of steroid injections, placement of stints or placement of flaps must be done. The location of the stenosis may be of importance when determining the proper laser treatment or combination of surgical interventions.

Polyps, Granulomas or Nodules can be treated with the laser, with vaporization and meticulous removal of all debris, Usually speech therapy and other post operative treatment, such as "stop smoking" is recommended for these patients. If there's questionable pathology, an excisional biopsy should be taken for histo-pathological examination.

Arytenoidectomy can successfully be managed with laser treatment. Vocal cord paralysis causes respiratory stridor and using the laser for this problem can avoid the need for permanent tracheostomy or an open laryngeal procedure. This procedure is done with the CO_2 laser attached to the microscope, using 400 mm objective lens and discreet ablation of the arytenoid body is carried out in a "hands-off" technique, in a vary narrow space.

The CO_2 laser and recently, the YAG laser with the synthetic sapphire contact probes, have been used in head and neck surgery. Since the laser beam seals the lymphatics and coagulates blood vessels during excision, the possibility of dissemination of malignant cells during the surgical procedure is reduced. If there's an infection at the planned operative site, it's not a contraindicate because, when the laser is used it sterilizes the tissue. There's usually no complication post operatively, blood loss is reduced and healing is comparable to conventional surgery. Also, there seems to be reduced edema and post operative pain is markedly deminished.

ON GOING MANAGEMENT of the patient having **Otolaryngolgical** procedures includes maintaining adequate airway, continually observing the patient for airway obstruction, maintaining adequate intake and output, and keeping the voice at rest by supplying materials such as a pad of paper or "magic-slate" for communication. For those patients having major head and neck procedures, the above post operative instructions should be prepared and instructions on the care of tracheostomy or laryngectomy tubes or stomas will be necessary.

The Perioperative Care of Patients

This will be post operative teaching for the patients and his/her family who will need emotional support, also. Explanation of all procedures provides encouragement for the patient and the family to return to independent living. The patient will need instruction on maintaining their diet, shielding the stoma during a shower, how to shave with a stoma; keeping the stoma covered, how to dress and the continued use of a humidifier, the signs of respiratory distress and the need to wear a medical alert device. The patient will need continued psycho-social support, referral to a home health agency and to understand the importance of patient care.

Aerodigestive Tract

Acute gastrointestinal bleeding is a common cause of hospital admissions and there's significant mortality despite recent advances in therapy. Many forms of non-surgical therapy have been advocated for such lesions. Notable numbers of patients, having exhausted all forms of medical therapy, continue to bleed and mortality is high, ranging to 35%. The last resort is surgery on a high risk patient in a try to control the hemorrhage.

With technical advances in endoscopy and the advent of flexible fiberoptics, laser phototherapy is among the new modalities used for coagulation. Early on, the Argon laser was coupled with a laser endoscope, but the energy needed to control gastric bleeding was beyond the limits of existing laser equipment. The Nd: YAG laser had a greater energy density; this laser heats a volume of tissue about three times larger, and results of a comparable study showed the YAG laser being superior to the Argon laser for photocoagulation in patients having severe upper gastrointestinal bleeding.

With the introduction of the "CONTACT" Nd: YAG laser surgery there have been decided improvements in the techniques on controlling gastric bleeding, using minimally invasive procedures. The stomach must be lavages with ice slush, until clear of all clots and residue. Using a large "ewald" gastric tube, the gastric contents are lavages until clear of clots and the contents slightly pink tinged. The gastroscope is passed into the stomach and bleeding sites identified. Using the flat contact probe, a *rosette* pattern may shrink the vessel, denaturizing the protein in the gastric mucosa and tamponades the bleeding site. Because lower power densities are used the risk of perforation, plume is minimal not obscuring the site as water or saline is used as coaxial cooling, the thermal-physical effects control the bleeding, scarring happens, and decreases most sequential events. This procedure may have limited use, but offers the opportunity to stabilize a high risk patient in preparation for a surgical procedure. Laser irradiation produced a greater reduction in bleeding from gastric erosions when compared to electrocautery.

The advantage of laser photocoagulation is that the tissue coagulation is superficial and localized. Tissue damage can accurately be predicted and there's no physical contact with the bleeding. However, efficacy of the use of the YAG laser in photocoagulation in intestinal hemorrhage has limits and the physician may have to resort to immediate surgery.

Laser photocoagulation in the aerodigestive tract has been used in may other procedures. As the technology has advanced, we see the advantage of using laser techniques for a variety of procedures, allowing for minimally invasive surgery to happen, offering the patients a treatment choice. Although the Argon and Non-Contact Nd: YAG laser treatments have been used with limited success in the gastrointerstinal tract, the arrival of **contact laser surgery** has increased the types of treatments that can be preformed, using flexible endoscopes. The physical differences using non-contact and contact YAG techniques have been described in earlier chapters of this book.

The following is a review of several procedures that can be done using the laser in the gastrointestinal tract:

HEREDITY HEMORRHAGIC LESIONS (OSLER-WEBER-RENDER DISEASE)

Identified by mucocutaneous lesion and recurrent G.I. bleeding, with or without family history. In many patients, bleeding may be slow, chronic or insidious and patient are usually maintained on long term oral iron replacement medication and occasional transfusion therapy.

New lesions can form ever. Chronic bleeding can be controlled by laser photoablation and appears to re-bleed less frequently. Multiple lesions can be treated in a single session, usually discharged the same or following day. Patients are N.P.O. for about 6-8 hours, on a fluid diet for 24 hours then can resume a normal diet and activities of daily living.

Angiodysplasia

These are vascular malformations that happen in the cecum and ascending colon and 25% of the cases seem to be associated with aortic vascular disease. Most of the patients are in the geriatric age group with other associated medical problems such as; Chronic Obstructive Pulmonary Disease or Chronic Heart Disease. These lesions tend to bleed and can be successfully controlled on endoscopic examination by photocoagulating the lesion with minimal complications.

Other procedures that can be done endoscopically with the laser are small **muosae tears, in the Mallory-Weiss Syndrome, Esophageal Varcies, and Gastric Ulcers** that bleed. There are few complications when using the laser as these patients are high risk for major operative procedures and can be controlled using photocoagulation until such a time as they're stable and can with stand a major procedure, if necessary.

Palliation of obstructing and recurring tumors, such as **esophageal cancer** using photoablation or excision can give the patient an opportunity for a better quality of life. Long term survival of these patients past five years, is unusual, despite treatment and is only about 5%. Early diagnosis is prime for curation using conventional or "standard" treatment. Patients often overlook early symptoms that may show primary carcinoma of the esophagus. Sore throats, often ignored as part of a cold or allergy, not being able to swallow, or just generally not feeling well, often attributed to the "flu" even with some weight loss is ignored until all the symptoms bring the individual to the physician, almost to late for long, successful treatment.

Patient selection is based on confirmed histological diagnosis, medical history; including any bleeding tendencies. Patients are at risk because of mal-nourishment often have a parentral nutrition series to improve their prognosis. Depending on the severity of the obstruction, the patient is maintained on a clear liquid diet for about 1-2 days before the laser procedure. The pre-operative preparation of the patient includes:

- Education of the patient to; understanding they'll have a large "tube" passed into their throat an may fell sore after the procedure.

- They may smell a noxious odor and have a "sour" taste in their mouth. They may also have halatosis 1-3 days post laser treatment.

- They'll have to wear protective eye wear if they're done under local anesthesia.

The equipment for this procedure isn't unlike most gastroenterology procedures, and they following should be available:

- Two channel gastroscope
- Light source
- Teaching scope or video monitor
- Biopsy and grasping forceps
- Attenuators for scope viewing window
- Esophageal dilators
- Suction for laser plume and secretions
- Smoke evacuation system

The procedure is usually done in the endoscopy suite. Patients have intravenous lines started the night before the procedure with incremental doses of anti-secretory drugs. Diazepam and Mepiridine given during the procedure to maintain the patient's discomfort level. The procedure, if done with non-contact YAG laser techniques are usually done under general anesthesia or I.V. Sedation with Anesthesia standby and in one to four settings, as the procedure uses air as a coolant.

The absorption of the laser energy into the tissue causes thermal necrosis, the heat distribution in intolerable to the patient over long periods of time. If the procedure is done using contact YAG laser procedures, the patient doesn't usually have general anesthesia but topical anesthesia potentiated with I.V. sedation.

The contact tip is cooled by a liquid solution and the absorption is tissue is less as there's decreased energy absorption in the surrounding tissue. The patient seen to tolerate the procedure and ablation of the tumor, depending on the size, can be done in one or two settings. When a significant lumen have been established the patient can be discharged however, there are several post laser discharge instructions for consideration, they are:

- Nutrition consultation. Often, patients will begin on hi-protein liquids and progress to a soft diet.
- Keeping, the lumen open may need return as an outpatient for esophageal dilation.
- The patient and family need to have access to cancer counseling groups.
- Understanding that recurring symptoms may need further laser ablation.

Complications from laser procedures may be perforation, causing esophageal-tracheal fistula; aspiration, pneumothorax, and there may be several days of expectoration of debris from the tumor ablation. Most complications are treated by conventional modalities. A major risk from retreated palliation is perforation of a major vessel that has become incorporated in the tumor mass. This is usually unpredictable and may cause death as the result of the procedure. Similar laser procedures can be applied to lower colonic tumors, either benign or malignant. These patients all need long term follow-up care and support.

Gynecology

Laser therapy in gynecology is divided into three groups; lower tract, endoscopic, and intra-abdominal procedures Most of the gynecologic work continues being done with the CO/2 laser, however, recently the Nd: YAG's laser's efficacy in this area has emerged. There's significant evidence in the literature that the Argon and Green only wavelength may have applications in certain gynecological procedures. The following discussion will concern the care of patients having procedures done with the CO/2 and Nd: YAG laser.

In most of the **lower tract** gynecologic procedures, the use of the laser has become the treatment of choice. Many procedures now being done with patients staying overnight are being done on an outpatient basis. The CO/2 laser used in the treatment of cervical intra-epitheal neoplasia (CIN) has predictable cure rates of to 97%, depending on the classification of the CIN. Other treatments are surgical and include; conization, cryotherapy or cautery, with cure rates of about 67%. A hysterectomy is the ultimate decision to resolve this disease process. Other lower tract gynecologic diseases treated with the CO/2 laser are lesions of the vulva, vagina, and cervix that include leukoplakia, condyloma, vaginal adenosis, vaginal warts and herpes. Many of these procedures are done with the laser attached to the microscope or culposcope. Because of the ease of using the laser in this area, many physicians may use the laser in their office practice.

How to treat diseases of the lower genital tract have plagued gynecologists since the early 1900's when many physiopathological diseases were being recognized by the process in the early stages. In 1932, several physicians worked together to define the pre-malignant stages of carcinoma in situ and the epitheal changes were described in 1962 at an International Cytology Meeting. In 1974, the laser was first used on CIN. In 1925, the culposcope was developed and gained quick acceptance for the use in gynecology. Now the laser mounted on a culposcope allows the gynecologist precision and a diagnostic tool that can be used to do microsurgery in the lower genital tract.

Although cold conization or cryotherapy has been the standard accepted method of treatment, there are several disadvantages such as; high percentage of recurrent disease, scarring, stenosis, cervical incompetence and post operative bleeding. The laser, however, can treat lesions large or small by excision, vaporization, or a combination of the two techniques, with precision under microscopic control.

Instruments, equipment and supplies needed are:

Equipment	• Lasers $CO/2$ or Nd: YAG • Microscope or culposcope • Smoke evacuator and tubing Instruments • D and C Set • Anal Set • Graves and Aavard Speculums • Straight and lateral calipers • #10 knife blade and handle • Cervical Block Tray
Medication	• 4% acetic acid • Lugols solution • Pitressin • 1% Lidocaine • Oxycel
Other Supplies	• 0 - Chromic suture on cutting needle • Long Swabs • Irrigating solution • Peri pads

The patient is usually in lithotomy position, not draped, as the potential of ignition of the material presents a high risk. The patient is covered properly to assure privacy. The prep is finished and the perineium dried (as prep solution contains a minimum of alcohol) a wet gauze, tampon or large cotton "plug" is placed in or over the rectum and secured by taping a towel across this area, unless the perianal area in incorporated in the surgical field. This prevents methane gas escaping and potential ignition and risks of perianal burns are avoided.

There are several laser procedures that can be done in this area besides, cervical conization. Others are of the vulva, vagina and perianal are for dysplasia, CIN, VIN, VAIN, genital warts, herpes, condyloma and hemorrhoidectomy. When the physician does these procedures the $CO/2$ laser is used and the power settings are between

25 to 50 watts, either in a continuous or pulsed mode. Depending on the focal length of the micro or culposcope, the spot size is usually 0.7 to 1.0 mm. If superpulse is used, these settings are changed significantly.

The Nd: YAG laser, using synthetic sapphire tips, can also be used to do these procedures. Micro or culposcopic identification of the pathology with conformation is necessary for cervical conization, vulvar or vaginal excisions; several hand pieces can be used; general, dental, or conization. This depends on the position or depth of the lesion. If the lesion is being excised a scalpel tip, either frosted or plain, is chosen. If vaporized, a round tip is used. The laser is set at 12-17 watts. Out lining borders are done in a pulsed mode and excision in continuous wave.

Immediate post operative instructions to the patient are:

- no douching except as ordered
- use only the medication prescribed
- no tampons, a sanitary pad is used
- no sexual intercourse for 2-3 weeks
- any bright red blood, call physician

There will be a slight bloody or serous discharge for one to three days, then a mild leukorrhea for five to seven days. Post operative hemorrhage is the major complication and happens within the first two weeks following the procedure. Most patients can be controlled by an application of silver nitrate to the area. Occasionally, a suture is needed to control the bleeding. There may be minor cramping, with any severe cramps or bleeding, the physician should be notified immediately. Follow-up visits to the physician should be at three to six weeks and at three to nine months, with both culposcopic and cytologic exams, especially for patients having histologic (CIN) cervical intra-epithelial neoplasia.

Post operative care for other lower tract gynecologic laser surgery includes; cleansing of the perineum three times a day, sitz bath or whirlpool, using a perineal lamp or hair dryer to keep the vulvar area dry, cleansing with witch hazel soaked cotton after urination and using oral analgesics if needed.

Post operative instruction after laser therapy for condylomata, vaginal warts and herpes include instructions; **not to have sexual intercourse for three weeks and then use condoms for three months or until** there's no proof of recurrence, to prevent sexual transmission of these diseases.

The use of endoscopes in gynecology has significantly reduced the intra-operative risk of open surgery and has reduce major operative procedures into minimally invasive procedures. The laparoscope and hysteroscope are chiefly used although, the use of the pelvoscope appears to have some merit.

Laser gynecological procedures began in late 1970 for laparoscopy and the early 1980's with the use of the hysterscope. The procedures currently being done are:

LAPAROSCOPIC	• Adhesions • Vaporization of Endometrosis • Neo-salpingostomy • Vaporization and excision small tumors • Ovarian cystectomy • Transection of utero-sacral ligments
HYSTEROSCOPIC	• Ablation endometrial lining • Vaporization/excision uteral septum • Uteral polyps • Transection of biconate uterus • Endo-cervical lesions

Equipment and supplies needed are:

LAPAROSCOPIC	• Laparoscopy tray • Verrus needle • Variable/high flow insufflator • Suction probes • Various grasping forceps and scissors • Quartz or titanium probes • Mono/bipolar cautery set-up • Fiber optic light source and cords • Two to four trocars with sleeves • Smoke evacuation system • Heprin solution for irrigation • #10 blade and knife handle • 2-0 Chromic suture on cutting needle • CO2 or Nd: YAG laser
HYSTEROSCOPIC	• D AND C SET • Biopsy forceps • Long and short scissors • Long and short probes • Hysterscopy instruments

- Fiber optic light source and cords
- Hank or Hagar dilators
- 2 3M (1016) irrigation pouches
- Heavy duty I.V. pole
- 3-5 3,000 cc bags of solution NACL or Ringers (not slush just cold)
- Large bore irrigation tubing
- 3-4 suction cannisters hooked in tandem
- Measuring pitcher (strict I and O)
- Nd: YAG laser and fiber with or with out contact tips

The technique for with procedure varies with how each surgeon has been trained. During laparoscopy procedures, the laser can be connected to the lens or various other puncture sites. The ancillary puncture sites may be for gas flow to maintain pneumoperitoneium or suction probes to manipulate tissue, smoke evacuation or irrigation. Maintaining a pneumoperitoneium is difficult as the CO2 laser creates much plume, but a trumpet valve on the suction line and a variable high rate flow insufflator have simplified the use of the laparoscope in the peritoneal cavity.

Some disadvantages of laser laparoscopy besides, difficulty maintaining laser alignment and visualizing the aiming beam is smoke accumulation obstructing visualization of tissue that may lead to injury to important intraperitoneal structures. Residual carbonization is irrigates with Ringers Solution and aspirated through one of the puncture sites.

Using the Nd: YAG laser with contact tips significantly reduces plume accumulation. Subsequently, the pneumoperitoneium is maintained longer without excessive insufflation. The round, chisel, or flat probe is used with the laparoscopy hand piece, depending on the procedure being done. Under direct vision the hysterscopy procedures are done with the Nd: YAG laser. Endometrial ablation, a new procedure for women having intractable benign bleeding, as an alternative to hysterectomy, need an in depth medical work-up, including biopsy of the uterine lining to define pathology and at least 30 days on Danocrine t^m to reduce or thin the endometrial lining. This procedure can be done with contact or non-contact technique and makes the uterine lining to scar, menses stop or decreases to a tolerable level. The patients having this procedure shouldn't be of child bearing age or want further children, as this procedure makes them sterile. Patient having endoscopy procedures are usually given a general anaesthetic and the procedures are done on an outpatient basis.

Post operatively, the laparoscopy patient may experience abdominal cramping and pain in the posterior shoulder area due to the high flow of the carbon dioxide gas used for insufflation during the procedure and may need minimal analgesics. Patients having hysteroscopy procedures need to be observed for symptoms of fluid overload because of the amount of fluid and rate of flow during this procedure. There may be some lower abdominal cramping and serous discharge post laser treatment, however, bleeding should be reported to the physician immediately.

Discharge instruction usually includes no heavy lifting. Report any discomfort or bleeding to the physician. If the endoscopy procedures are done for infertility, the prognosis alternatives, benefits and risks must be discussed with the patient and her partner.

Intra-abdominal gynecologic laser procedures include vaporization of endometrosis, myomectomy, debulking large tumors and infertility surgery. The use of the CO_2 laser in these procedures provides precision needed to vaporize endometriotic implants, reduces scarring, seals lymphatics and small blood vessels when used for incision, reducing blood loss and serous fluid in the pelvis which in turn reduces potential adhesions and increases the success rate in tubal reconstruction.

The Nd: YAG with the synthetic sapphire contact tips are also being used for a variety of procedures intra-abdominally. Similarly, to the CO_2, however, with much less plume accumulation. Although laser plume is reduced with the use of the contact tips, smoke evacuation should be done for good visualization of the operative site. The contact tips used in intra-abdominal gynecology surgery are; frosted or plain scalpels, chisel tips or round probes on general surgery handpieces, depending on the procedure. The laser power settings are between 10-20 watts, continuous wave mode. The use of the contact laser methods gives the physician tactile feedback and precision, especially when lysing adhesions and debulking large tumors.

Smoke evacuation systems are important for the evacuation of the laser plume during cases of known or suspected viral diseases. Using the laser to vaporize, ablate and excise these lesions have a documentated cure rate of about 95%. There's increased concern whether there's viable particulate matter in laser plume.

Viral lesions of the external genitalia, both male and female has increased with the current sexual attitudes, today. Current smoke evacuation systems are very effective if the plume is evacuated close

The Perioperative Care of Patients 119

to the point of origin as possible. Special Filters must be used if the internal vacuum system is used. Laser particulate matter is about 0.3 microns, double masking filters about 80% of the particulate matter and allows breathe-ability. New masks and smoke evacuators systems are on the market and seem more efficient. All disposable items are disposed of following the facilities procedure for bio-hazard material. All equipment is washed with anti-microbial solution, laser instruments and other accessories are decontaminated and sterilized using the standard methods for the instruments used.

Practical consideration for the nurse, when dealing with women who has histo-pathological problems needing laser surgery, is understanding the effect of the pathology or diagnosis to the patient and her family. Typically, these patients have high anxiety and emotional reactions either resulting from infertility, a sexually transmitted disease or pre-invasive cancer. Her reactions to the diagnosis and recommended treatment events will depend on her attitude to herself, sexuality and the relationship with her partner. Patient education information is helpful and the opportunity should be afforded for interactive participation with the health care provider. As many laser procedures are done on an outpatient basis, pre-operative assessment and instructions are important before admission and reinforcement at the time of admission. If the patient is done under local anaesthetic, her senses will be heightened, so there are many point of discussion that should happen with the clinical nurse regarding the laser interventional procedure, they are:

- There will be a noxious smell, her flesh being vaporized or excised.
- She may have a warm sensation from the thermal injury to tissue but shouldn't feel any discomfort.
- If the procedures becomes painful to notify the physician immediately.
- She will have to eye protection of the correct optical density for the laser used.
- She will hear sound of machinery, the laser and the smoke evacuator.
- She will need to be assured her privacy will be maintained always.

The nurse should be ready to discuss honestly, the effect of sexually transmitted diseases with the patient as many pose a continuing social dilemma. The time taken with the patient in helping her to understand the expected outcomes of her laser intervention will ally the fears and reaction of the disease process and reduce the long term psycho-social effects for the patients, her partner and family. It'll be of utmost importance that the nurse treat her patient with honest, fair and trusting attitudes to aid the patient in accepting her disease process as many of these patients need long term follow-up care.

Discharge instruction should include an explanation of the importance of; the medications regimes, abstaining from sexual intercourse or douching until indicated by the physician, avoid sitting for long periods prevent venous stasis, avoiding constipation, reporting vaginal bleeding or severe cramping immediately and shouldn't do any heavy lifting for about six to eight weeks. The patient should be given an opportunity to verbalize her concerns and be encouraged to participate in follow-up care.

Urology

Laser used in urologic procedures include; CO_2, Argon and Nd: YAG systems. The CO_2 laser is used for external procedures such as; penile warts, condyloma and partial peniectomy for tumors. The Argon laser, because of its limited necrosis and ability to be used with fiberoptics, is used in urethral and bladder papillomas. Recently, the Nd: YAG laser has become a treatment of choice for transuretheral resection of bladder tumors, to include contact laser surgery and with the contact tips for open procedures such as; partial nephrectomies or orchidectomy. Some physicians have begun to use the contact techniques for adult circumcisions.

Clinical application of lasers in urology have increase and currently lesions of the external genitalia and internal genitourinary system are done with lasers as a choice to conventional procedures. As urology is currently using three laser wavelengths many procedures have become minimally invasive and have reduced the patients length of stay in the hospital or have become out patient procedures. There's reduced bleeding, scarring, post operative discomfort and sometimes no foley catheters will be needed for long term irrigation. The Argon and Nd: YAG laser wavelengths pass through clear fluid and can be done under local anesthesia. Instruments used for these procedures are the generally used cystoscopes and panendoscopes, flexible ureteroscopes, guide wires, laser albarans bridge, dilators and laser fibers and contact tips and hand pieces where applicable. The technique using the laser depends on where the disease is located. In the bladder, non-contact YAG laser fibers, with the laser set at 50 watts with pulse durations of 4 seconds and with contact tips, usually the

The Perioperative Care of Patients

round or chisel tips are chosen, the YAG laser is set at 15-20 watts, continuous wave and pulse mode can be picked. Uretheral strictures may need post laser stints being inserted. Vaporization of lesions in the meatus or ureter cause minimal tissue damage, reducing post operative stricture, scarring and often the need for repeated dilatations.

Patients having intra-abdominal laser procedures post operative care isn't unlike what we'd expect with conventional surgery, they're; encourage the patient to ambulate early, insure adequate intake and output, provide incisional support when coughing and deep breathing, use mild laxatives, as needed, and check the incision site for signs of infection. If the laser is used to make the incision, as it tends to seal the lymphatics, there may be some delay in wound healing and the stitches or skin clips should stay in the incision longer to prevent dehiscence.

Lesions of the external genitalia include condyloma, penile warts, adult circumcisions, Pyronies disease, or cancer. The wavelengths that can be used are the CO2 and contact Nd: YAG laser techniques. The microscope is particularly useful to inspect the area for more lesions. For condyloma and penile warts the CO2 laser in a defocused mode about 5-8 watts, in a continuous wave or pulsed mode is used. The areas are prepped in the usual fashion and the procedure can be done under local or general anesthesia. The area is washed with 3-4% **acetic acid** to identify the lesions, the char is washed off with saline or hydrogen peroxide and surface ablation is carried out aver all lesions. Post laser treatment the patient is instructed to apply **sulfidine creme** to the lasered areas. If all lesions are identified and have laser therapy, only about 5% of the patient will have recurrent lesions. Carcinoma of the penis is usually associated with mutilative surgery, using the CO2 or contact YAG lasers, control of the disease may have cosmetic results better to conventional amputative surgery. Bleeding is controlled and there's minimal post operative discomfort.

There's limited instrumentation for these procedures, as the lesion is excised or ablated with laser energy. A minor or plastic set may be needed especially for the penile carcinoma procedures. Smoke evacuation has been described earlier in this chapter and it's recommended that these procedures be followed for urological laser procedures.

Post operative care for external laser therapy of condyloma and penile warts are the same as the care given to women for the same procedures. Patient having Argon or YAG laser treatment for bladder papilloma or tumors are now being treated on an out patient basis. Because the laser is used in a fluid medium the heat from the laser energy is disapated, so the patient may feel warmth but shouldn't be uncomfortable. There's little or not post operative bleeding and usually a foley catheter and bladder irrigation isn't necessary. Post operative care for patients having internal bladder laser procedures call for them to increase their fluids, refrain for drinking alcohol for 3-7 days post operative reducing the probability of a bleeding episode, and report and bright red bleeding immediately to the physician, there may be some mild hematuria for a couple of days. Patients will have follow-up care on an out patient basis.

General Surgery

Although, the CO_2 laser was generally used first by many general surgeons for a variety of procedures such as; debulking of intra-abdominal tumors, tries at liver resections, lysis of adhesions, vaporization of various skin lesions and hemorrhoidectomies, it wasn't well received by this speciality. Most General Surgeons felt they could do these procedures as well with the knife, and their conventional techniques so they became skeptical about the efficacy of lasers in general surgery.

Somewhat successful, as it reduces blood loss when it was used, especially where there were small blood vessels and the lymphatic were sealed, especially in oncologic surgery. Again, as it was a no-touch-technique, the CO2 laser wasn't generally accepted as general surgeon depend on touching tissues to guide them as they do the various procedures. Since the advent of the synthetic sapphire contact tips, used as scalpels, giving the surgeons tactile feedback, is beginning to look as good a tool for the general surgeons. Now the Nd: YAG laser is used as a "light knife" and becoming an accepted modality in general surgery for a variety of procedures. The advantages are:

- Reduced blood loss
- Minimal tissue damage
- Reduced post operative discomfort
- Reduced length of stay
- Minimally invasive procedures
- Out patient procedures
- Return of tactile feedback for surgeon

The procedures most commonly done by the general surgeons with the laser are; mastectomy, either or both radical or modified, cholecystectomy, hernia repairs, especially if a flap or mesh repairs is needed, intra-abdominal procedures such as debulking of tumors, liver and pancreatic resections, extrinsic tumors of the bowel and lysis of adhesions. The colon-rectal surgeons are using the same laser system for hemorrhoidectomy, anal fissures or fistulas and anal warts or condyloma.

The instrumentation for these procedures aren't unlike those used when doing conventional procedures, the following is a like of instrument that should have a matte' or none shinny finish.

- Hemostats
- Right Angles
- Babcocks
- Allis Forceps
- Titanium Backstops
- Retractors
- Anal Scopes
- Vascular Clamps
- Tissue Forceps
- Bowel Clamps

It's unnecessary to have a separate "Laser Pan" and these instruments can be used during conventional surgery.

Other equipment will be the Nd: YAG laser, and depending on the type of procedure, a general surgery or dental hand piece, with a variety of contact tips and scalpels available. All safety rules are followed; eye protection of the correct optical density, smoke evacuation system, viewing windows covered and the procedure documented.

Because the laser fiber is fragile verify that it's secured to the field however, do **NOT** string it under the mayo stand or use sharp instruments. It's best held together in a folded towel. Often, a fiber will be broken or dropped during the procedure when the first calibration is complete, it's recommended that two calibrations sleeves be sterilized for recalibration, if needed.

The contact tips and calibration sleeves can be steamed sterilized at 270°F on a 3 minute flash cycle before each procedure. An **institutional** policy can be developed regarding the re-sterilization of fibers and handpieces, being reused. Many institutions use the resterilized fibers on cases such as hemorrhoidectomies, condyloma, or rectal tumors. If the resterilization process is approved these accessories can be sterilized in ethylene oxide on the cool cycle and airated for 12 hours. These products can be bought unsterile as requested.

Post operative care of these patients are the same as the care for those patients having major intra-abdominal surgery with or without the laser. There may be two added benefits in using the laser; (1) less post operative infection, has been reported as it's theorized that the laser energy sterilized the tissue. Several studies have been done on patients having laser resection of infected decubitus ulcers with a known cultured bacteria and after the laser procedure the bacteria counts have been significantly reduced. And (2) although, it's difficult to quantitate and is subjective, most laser patients seem to have reduced post operative discomfort and need minimal or no analgesics.

There are other post operative considerations and suggestions for discharge instruction for those patients having general surgical procedures, they are:

MASTECTOMY; when having an axillary dissection the patient should have the axilla packed with fluffs and a chest binder or ace wrap comfortably holding the dressing in place, for about two day toprevent seroma formation. Usually, on the second post operative day these patients can begin the "Reach-To-Recovery" program. You will note decreased drainage and little need for analgesics and many patient are discharged on the third post operative day; unless they have other medical problems.

CHOLECYSTECTOMY with or without a common duct exploration is done through a smaller incision with little or no blood loss. The gall bladder is dissected from the liver bed with the laser and usually needs no liver suture. Patients who has a common duct exploration may need a T-Tube, however, penrose drains are rarely used if the procedure is done with the laser. Patients have little post operative discomfort and depending on age; severity of illness or other complicating medical factors patients are usually discharges between 2-4 days post operatively. Average length of stay forcholecystectomies is 3-5 days, longer with other medical complications affect the patients recovery.

HERNIA with or without mesh repair. The laser offers the surgeon to raise a flap for the mesh repair with little or no bleeding. These patient usually stay less than 2 days post operatively. Hernia repairs without mesh repair can be done on an outpatient basis, should they have no other complicating medical problems. Many patients may prefer to stay on the short stay unit (24 hours) until they urinate and feel comfortable walking. These patients tolerate early ambulation, with little discomfort needing minimal post operative analgesia.

HEMORRHOIDECTOMY, AND OTHER ANAL PROCEDURES done with the laser are now done as outpatients. If the Nd: YAG and contact laser surgery technique is used discharge instructions will be important. The following information should be included:

- Keep area dry and clean using sitz bath with "ocean water," pat dry and apply witch hazel pads for comfort.
- The use of a maxi or mini sanitary pad that sticks to the under pants with an adhesive strip maintains cleanliness

- and reduces embarrassment and can easily be changed and discarded. **Note;** Male patients may need a demonstration on how to use this product.

- If the patient cannot void before discharge, they are catheritized, with instruction on what to do if this happens when they're home.

- Any bleeding is immediately reported to the physician and if he's not readily available the patient should be instructed to return to the emergency room.

- Patients are usually put on a high fiber, low roughage diet and a stool softener for several weeks to prevent painful bowel movements and straining post operatively.

INTRA-ABDOMINAL patients having their procedures with the laser will need to ambulate early, cough and deep breath or have respiratory therapy, diet as tolerated, and they may be on praental therapy and the intravenous site will need to be checked frequently and the dressing and site change according to hospital policy.

There are few post operative complication when the laser has been used during the procedure. However, patients need to be aware that the laser is a surgical tool and the energy must be delivered to the target tissue and that usually mean an incision. Sometimes such as; rectal polyps or tumors, gastric bleeding, and other gastrointestinal indications, instead of a major surgical procedure, these surgical indications may convert to a minimally invasive procedure and be done with the laser through a flexible endoscope.

The specialty of general surgery although slow to use the laser now, with the ability to have tactile feedback using the contact tips, are beginning to realize the advantages of using the laser; giving their patients increased quality care.

DERMATOLOGY AND PLASTIC SURGERY

The specialties of Dermatology and Plastic Surgery overlap, also, Facial Plastics that the Otolaryngologists are now including in their specialty. When laser procedures were introduced into medicine and surgery outside Ophthalmology the Dermatologists saw the efficacy of the visible wavelengths for the pigmented lesions. Both the CO_2 and Argon-ion lasers are used in these specialties for a variety of lesions, they can be ablated, vaporized, or excised. Theoretically, the laser seals the lymphatics preventing the dissemination of malignant cells, seals the vascular bed, and the thermal energy appears to sterilize the surgical field. The surgeon must assess the type of lesion being removed and choose the proper wavelength. Tattoos can be vaporized, or ablated using either the CO2 or Argon-ion laser. The tattoo is never removed as there's scarring, and the physician must take care not to leave "ghosting" when trying to remove the tattoo. The Nd: YAG laser with the contact tips has recently entered this specialty, particularly for the use of vascular tumors. All the current laser wavelengths used in medicine and surgery have application for procedures of the skin, especially in the head and neck area where there are small blood vessels.

Patients having Keloid lesions are extremely difficult to treat, by all standard methods and surgical techniques tend to have recurrence of the lesion, frequently to a greater extent. Several centers have worked on Keloids with the CO2 laser and have found improved wound healing with minimal re-scarring and less pain, the use of intra-lesional steroids are recommended. Other lesions that respond with the used of the CO2 laser are; plantar and other types of warts, papillomas, kertosis, angiosarcoma, rhinophyma and many other lesions of the dermal and epidermal layers of the skin.

The set up for most of these procedures is:

- Local, regional or general anesthesia
- Prep with desired solution and pat dry
- Drape in normal fashion, area around lesion wet
- Plastic instrument tray
- Lasers can be:
  - CO2 using handpieces or micromanipulator
  - Argon-ion using collimated handpiece
- Smoke evacuation system
- Eye protection of the correct optical density
- Irrigation fluid
- Dressings and ointment or medication as needed

Most patients have regional or local anesthesia and should have preoperative education to reduce their anxiety and increase their understanding of the procedure. As these patients are awake and explanation of how the laser is used and the surgical environment including; eye wear, smoke evacuation and other nursing duties that will happen.

Post operatively these patients must be taught meticulous wound care techniques to prevent anyf infection. Cleansing the wound twice a day with mild soap and water or a mild anti-bacterial solution, followed

The Perioperative Care of Patients

by an application of an antibiotic ointment (physician preference), covered by a light dressing, is continued until healing has occurred. The keloids may need a pressure dressing to deter hypertrophic Complication using the CO2 laser range between 1-4%, and mainly fall into two categories, infection or hypertrophic scarring. Other complications can be; bleeding, granulation of tissue, unexpected pain or prolonged healing.

The Argon-ion laser, with its wavelength having preferential absorption by hemoglobin, is useful for the destruction of vascular and pigmented lesions. When laser energy is delivered to the lesion there's preferential absorption, limited dermal injury, and subsequent fibroblastic response. When vascular injury and thrombosis are minimal, the desirable result is marked lightening of pigmented lesions without scarring. The pigmented lesions can be hemoglobin, melanin, or suspended pigments of tattoo or foreign body particles causing a controlled burn to the superficial layers of the skin, similar to a 2nd o burn. The necrotic tissue sloughs and is replaced by new, thin pink epithelial tissue. Portwine Stains (PWS) before laser surgery had no other effective treatment. Usually, occurring on the face, followed by incidences on the trunk, neck upper and lower extremities. After the treatment with the Argon-ion laser there seems to be a lightening effect and continue to improve for up to 2 year.

Nursing involvement with patients that have laser therapy for pigmented lesions, particularly on the face and neck, begins by helping the patient to cope with the psycho-social affect of these lesions on his/her self concept and work with the patient and family to understand the disease process and long term therapy that may be needed. These patients will be outpatients and have multiple laser treatments for large pigmented lesions. Local anesthesia in injected and the eyes are protected with safety glasses or covered with stainless steel eye cups after a mild topical anesthesia is instilled in the eye. The nurse gives continued support throughout the laser procedure.

Post operative care is continues, as the patient may return for additional laser treatments. Basic wound care is taught to prevent infection. Immediately, post operatively, the patient may feel dizzy which is thought to be a vagal response. Patients are encouraged to be involved in their treatment and encouraged to look at the area treated before it's bandaged. The skin reaction that will follow is a response to a predictable pattern and the patient is constantly reminded to adhere to simple wound care to achieve satisfactory results. The patient is encouraged to continue their treatment and outpatient care.

Discharge instructions for patients having their Portwine Stains ablated with the Argon-ion laser are:

- Sleep with the bed elevated to reduce edema
- Ice bags to treated area decreases edema and pain
- Wound care until "weeping" ends and "scab" forms
  - wash gently with ivory or basic soap rinse well
  - pat dry, use hair dryer on low
- Apply prescribed antibiotic ointment, very thin
- Cover with dressings as instructed

NOTE: Remove dressings carefully as to not interrupt healing, if the seem "stuck" soak in warm water.

Wound care after healing (scab) forms:
- Keep area clean using mild soap
- Ointment can be discontinued
- WOMEN: Make-up can be applied, lightly
- MEN: Can shave when healed completely
- Other general instructions:
  - Avoid exposure to direct sunlight
  - Aspirin containing products to be avoided
  - Use Tyenol™, Advil™, Nuprin™ for pain
- Report any bleeding, redness, elevated temperature, to the physician, immediately.

As laser therapy is accepted in all disciplines of medicine and surgery, new surgical procedures will be developed, and all nurses will need to update their knowledge bases as this technology is introduce to their practice. This chapter on the perioperative role and nursing interventions have been the attempt to meet the need to assess, plan, implement the nursing care plan, evaluate the outcomes and understand the risks associated with laser technology as we give quality patient care.

SUMMARY

The nurse will play a major role during laser practice in medicine and surgery as the technology proliferates in health care facilities. Nursing practice during laser procedures isn't essentially different from the conventional surgical routine for that procedure. Essential is the basic understanding of laser biophysics, the effect of the laser on tissue; advantages of the laser as a surgical tool, and the impact new technology will have on their daily practice. Pre operative assessment is similar to that for all other surgical interventions. The patient may have increased anxiety about the use of the laser during the surgical procedure, this may be increased because of the public exposure to lasers in science fiction media. The simple explanation of the procedure and the advantages of using the laser allays these fears. Intra-operative plans call for operational understanding of the laser systems and related accessories, instrumentation and laser safety requirements. Post operative care and evaluation don't deviate from the normal post operative care for conventional surgical procedures. The most common difference appears to be reduce post operative discomfort, less need for analgesics, and reduced length of stay in the hospital. Many laser procedures can be done on an outpatient basis, where some procedures might have been major procedures often they're minimally invasive procedures when done with the laser. Most laser procedures are done in a cost effective delivery of health care to the consumer as the laser is an additional tool added to the physicians armamentarium that gives him/her another option as a treatment choice.

CHAPTER 12
THE FUTURE...

"If we could see beyond today... " what's on the horizon in laser therapy? We hear " buzzwords " like; double frequency YAG, Excimer, Metal Vapor, CO2 fibers, Holmium, Nd: YLF, photodynamic therapy, and FEL (free electron lasers)! How does this impact the operating room and the support staff? " Dream " lasers, not yet available would look like medical gas columns, whatever wavelength needed, reach up, remove the laser fiber from the column, connect to an optical coupler, call the laser control room and ask for the wavelength, power, and mode and ZAP! To make these dream lasers come true will take intense research, a significant amount of money and acceptance by the medical community. Will all surgical interventions use the laser? Probably not, however by the year 2000, the laser has potential to become a standard tool in the operating room.

The future in now; oncology, cardiovascular, peripheral vascular, orthopedics, pediatrics, biostimulation, acupuncture (pain control) and holography doing three dimensional x-rays or body scans, the enormous potential of the use of laser in medicine and surgery is only limited by current technology and the user's mind.

Currently, in oncology, another adjunctive modality is being tried for clinical application, with the use of a variety of injectable dyes that respond at a photochemical level can be used to treat a variety of cancers. Endogenous porphyrins, constituents of hemoglobin, have been injected in tumor cells and when exposed to ultra-violet light give off a red-orange fluoresence. In 1972, Dr. Thomas Dougherty and his colleagues began experiments with a hematoporphyrin derivative and various light systems and wavelengths.

They found that although there was reaction to wavelengths at 414-517 nm that red light at 633 nm, penetrated the tissue and when used with hematoporphyrin derivative, causes a photochemical reaction that produces singlet oxygen and causes the tumor cells to necrosis. Newer sensitizers are being researched that are enhanced by other wavelengths, such as 1064 nm, in a pulsed mode.

How do these work? The patient receives a bolus injection of about 2.5 to 3 milligrams per kilogram of body weight of the photosensitizer. The photosensitive dye disseminates throughout the body, moving out of normal cells but staying longer in tumor cells. In about 48-72 hours after the injection the patient is exposed to 633 nm of laser light, causing a photochemical reaction and tissue death. Why the laser?

Other light sources are inefficient and can't be directed or focused directly to the source, especially to various sites in the body. The laser light can be optically pumped through fiberoptics and passed through a variety of endoscopes to reach the site of the tumor. Since there's less dye in the normal tissue, less severe or no tissue reaction happens. Some newer photosensitizers are absorbed quickly in tumor tissue and are excreted through the kidneys in about 12 hours. The tumor cells retain the "dye" and treatment can be give earlier.

Currently, this method is investigational and not a miraculous cure-all, but for selective patients, can be an adjunctive therapy when other therapies have been tried. Patients who agree to have this type of therapy must receive specific instructions as they become very photosensitive for about 20-45 day. They'd be instructed to keep all body parts out of direct sunlight especially those parts uncovered during normal, daily activity. Close their blinds or shades during the day and try to do outside errands in the evening or night. Even after the extend time of photosensitivity, to wear a sunscreen when outside and go outside in short, sequences until they can be assured there's no more photosensitivity. The major complication to this treatment is like a 2-3 o sunburn. It's clearly a challenge to the medical researchers and the related fields of biochemistry to find better answers for this therapy.

Another area in laser therapy is the use of a pulsed laser on caculi, all types. Depending, on the physical composition of the caculi they could be fragmented by the impact of laser energy. The short pulsed tunable dye laser at 577 nm has recently be approved for this process and concurrent reach is continuing with out caculi that can be formed in the patients body.

The laser at 577 nm is also being used in Dermatology and Plastic Surgery as it emits a "yellow" color that's absorbed is brown pigment and show promise in some the skin lesions.

Laser research in the vascular, both cardio and peripheral have enjoyed an intense interest and major response to prove that lasers are being used efficaciously in these area. There are several medical research projects that have been brought into the clinical arena for use, especially in the peripheral vascular system. A variety of wavelengths are being used from Argon-ion, Nd: YAG to Excimer and many still in the experimental stage. A variety of associated equipment is being developed simultaneously, such as; angioscopes, steerable catheters and other delivery systems. There has been F.D.A. approval for an Argon-ion system and many centers are doing laser-assisted balloon angioplasty in the operating room or interventional radiology. The

Argon laser will heat a metal tip that opens the blocked lumen. In the United States, Austria, France and Japan, the use of the sapphire tips and the YAG laser has been introduced with some success. In the United States and Canada the Excimer laser has been used expermentally in the clinical setting. Other lasers have received the I.D.E. to begin clinical experimentation in the vascular specialties, to open "clogged" arteries.

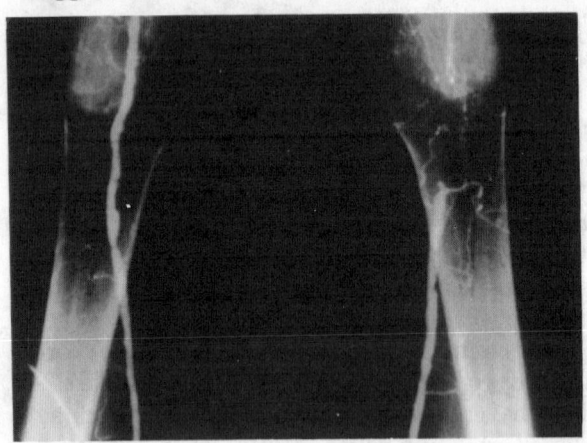

Figure 12.1
Laser Assisted Angioplasty

The use of lasers in Orthopedics is around the corner, although several physicians have been doing research with the CO2 laser for about four years and in the last two years the contact laser methods are making some head way, particularly in arthroscopy. There have been articles in the literature describing the use the CO2 laser to remove "bone cement" during a redo total hip. However, evacuation of the noxious fumes that happen when the methyl-methacrylate is exposed to the laser energy, presents a major problem.

With the advent of the synthetic sapphire tips the use of the Nd: YAG laser is being evaluated during menisectomy and patella procedures. Also, this laser system is being used during a variety of plastic hand procedures done in orthopedics. The contact techniques is currently being used for soft tissue incision, to reduce blood loss.

The application of low-output lasers being used in tissue "welding" is being studied, using microvascular techniques, as the protein is denaturized a bonding happens with the tissue and an anastomosis is formed. This technique could potentially be used in vasucular, nerves,

The Future

vas defrens and other possible anastomosis of tubular structures. This technique, experimentally, appeared to have superior wound healing at the site of the anastomosis.

Other uses for low-output lasers are being researched in the field of biostimulation. Among these experiments the physicians are looking for enhanced wound healing. Preliminary results suggest that low energy lasers may be useful for the enhancement of collagen deposits in a chronic necrotic process, such as; leg ulcers, decubiti, keloids and hypertrophic scarring.

Other new technology for medical lasers is being introduced in may specialties. The Double-Frequency Nd: YAG laser, that emits a wavelength of pure green light at 532 nm and has a clinical tissue effect close to the Argon laser is used in otolaryngology, gynecology and urology and in being introduce to Dermato-Plastic procedures. Currently, very costly technology, however, can be direct through a variety of fiberoptic endoscopes, is in the visible wavelength, and has minimal absorption in hemoglobin and oxyhemoglobin, minimal absorption in clear fluid; making it a valuable tool for non-invasive intra-ocular procedures. There are also other harmonics of YAG being investigated for use in medicine and surgery.

Another development in laser technology is a laser that can deliver two wavelength through the same machine, and use either and articulated arm or fiberoptics, and either wavelength in sequence or simultaneously. This type of unit, although very large and bulky would save space in the operating room and could be dedicated and all the laser procedures done in the same room; this reduces the flexibility of using the laser efficiently. There are several of these lasers in community hospitals.

There are newer wavelengths entering the medical field; Excimer lasers in the ultra-violet wave lengths. This laser uses an excited dimer, a noble gas such as Argon, Krypton or Xenon Fluoride and have wavelengths at 193, 248, and 351 nm's, respectively. These wave lengths can cause photo-chemical, thermal or acoustic effects are predictable for micro-surgical applications. The Excimer laser has been introduced in cardiovascular and ophthalmology.

Other lasers are; Metal Vapor lasers that emit wave lengths in the visible spectrum and could be used in Dermatology or Photodynamic Therapy. Other lasers being investigated use laser spectroscopy, scanning obstructions in the vascular system, sending that information to the computer and choosing the proper wavelength the ablate the lesion.

The role of the peri-operative nurse will continue to expand as new technology and laser applications proliferate in the medicine and surgery. Many questions are being raised regarding the standard of care, informed consent and other legal issues. Whoever will be setting the standards, surely the medical professional will be working with the laser specialist to define the laser treatment standards, safety aspects, and credentialing policies.

The cost effectiveness of laser procedures will affect reimbursement issues facing health care, today. It's incumbent upon the nursing profession to participate in developing the use of laser therapy that will be applicable to our nursing practice.

Issues of informed consent didn't change because the laser is being used as a treatment modality. However, although the patient may not fully comprehend all the physical properties of laser technology, the physician should explain in lay terminology, the nature if the procedure, what the laser is expected to complete, the significant risks, associated benefits, available choice of treatment and the expected outcomes. The essence of the informed consent doctrine is that the discussion happened between the physician and patient and the patient agrees to the procedure. Other legal issues will be addressed continually as the application of medical laser technology moves into the "mainstream" of generally accepted treatment modalities.

What does the future hold for the peri-operative nurse as the laser is introduce in her daily practice? The peri-operative nurse must continue to seek the knowledge to maintain an understanding of the laser in medicine and surgery, to participate in developing nursing standards about patients having laser procedures and continue to keep abreast of this fast-paced technology. The future is **now;** to this end this book is dedicated!

SUMMARY

What's the future of laser technology as it's applied to medicine and surgery? Surely, it's new technology, new delivery systems, not only technological but the way health care may be given eventually. Many questions are being raised regarding the efficacy of laser treatments in all area of medical and surgical practice. It's exciting be to at the leading edge of breakthroughs in patient care, but we the patient advocate must be ready to meet the challenges of the future. Nurses, must keep up with new and exciting innovations in medicine and surgery that affect their practice. The role of the peri-operative laser nurse is on the horizon of expanded practice. Nurses are becoming involved in collaborative practices with physicians developing education information for patients and their peers, implementing standards of care that affect health care delivery today. Nurses must be challenged to accept responsibility for quality care given to their patients in the 21 st. century.

Appendix

Appendix

APPENDIX

GLOSSARY

LASER TERMINOLOGY

Ablation	removal of tissue similar to cutting
Absorption	diffusion of radiation into thetissue with resultant energy transfer
Absorption Coefficient	wavelength's capability to be absorbed i.e.; in water or a point at which maximum energy is absorbed
Active Medium	the pumped medium that createshe laser light Aiming beam helium neon laser that has a red beam, coaxial with the laser being used
Amplitude	maximum height of each wave as it passes through a medium
Argon-ion	gas used as a laser medium
Attenuation	a decrease in the strength of light as it passes through a medium
Basic mode	usual (gaussion) profile of laser beam intensity
Carbon Dioxide	gas used as a laser medium, at 10600 nm and in the infrared range
Chromophere	content of tissue, i.e.; hemoglobin, melanin, keratin, water or protein
Coagulation	process known as clotting
Coherence	all waves are exactly in step (phase) with one another in both space and time
Continuous mode	consistent delivery of the laser beam equal to power density
Collimation	the laser beams are parallel with one another
Dichrotic filter	filter that allows some wavelengths to pass and not others
Dosimetry	amount of laser energy pumped into tissue
Electron	a negatively charged particle present in all atoms

Electromagnetic spectrum	frequencies and wavelengths given off by the atomic system
Endoscope	an instrument that can be inserted into the body so the physician can look inside. Flexible endo scopes are made out of fiberscopes and can be bent around corners.
Energy	Watts x Time = Joules
Energy source	high voltage electricity or intense flashes of light used to excite the laser medium
Excited State	atom with electrons in higher energy states
Excimer (excited dimer)	substances being used as the basis of lasers emitting ultra-violet light
External Power Source	a system outside the laser chamber that excites the photon
Femtoseconds	10 to the $^{-15}$ seconds
Fiberoptics	hundreds or even thousands of individual fibers are used totransmit laser light during treatment
Fluence	joules x centimeters squared
Focus/focal point	the exact point at which the laser waves are at peak power
Gaussian Curve	the cross section of radiant power density
Hemostasis	any procedure that stops bleeding
Hematopotphryin Derivative	a drug that is used inphotoradiation therapy and can be activated by laser light at 633 nm.
Joule	unit of energy
L.A.S.E.R.	Acronym for Light Amplification by the Stimu lated Emission of Radiation
Laser	a device that emits intense and power at close range, converting various frequencies of light in tosmall and extremely unified beam of one wave length of radiation
Laser Beam	energy source emanating from the laser
Laser Medium	a selected substance capable of giving rise to a laser source

Laser Terminology

Micromanipulator	a device that controls laser beam direction when connected to a microscope
Microprocessor	silicon chip computer that monitors and controls the operation of the laser
Mode	describes how the power of a laser beam is distributed within the beam
Mode-locked	laser wave output locked leaving the laser cavity in a controlled train of extreme short pulses
Monochromatic	waves are all the same length
Nd:YAG	Neodymium: Yttrium-Aluminum-Garnet, a crystal substance used as a laser medium
Nanometer	on nanometer is equal to 10 to the $^{-9\text{th}}$ meter this is the unit that wavelengths are often expressed
Nanosecond	is 10 to the $^{-9\text{th}}$ seconds
Optical Breakdown	at high energies the distribution of atoms freing electrons andforming a plasma shield
Optical Cavity	where the lasing medium isheld and excited
Output Coupler	the partially reflective mirror that allows a portion of the laser light to escape from the optical cavity
Phase / in phase	all the troughs and peaks coincide with each other. The result is a reinforced wave with an increase amplitude
Photocoagulation	the use of the laser beam to heat tissue below the vaporization level to coagulate tissue
Photon	unit of light energy
Plasma Shield	type of screen that uses energy to cause photodisruption or photothermolysis
Population Inversion	a state in which a substance has been energized so that more atoms or molecules are in a given excited state, this is necessary condition for laser action to occur
Power Density	the amount of energy concentrated into a spot of a particular size, and is expressed in watts per square centimeter

Pumping	process of supplying energy to the laser medium
PDT	photodynamic therapy, uses a dye that is injected into the patient and is selectively absorbed in tumor cells, when wavelengths of 514-630 nm are directed to the source, causes singlet oxygen to occur and tissue necrosis
Pulse	a discontinuous burst of laser light
Q-switched	employs a "quality" switching or shutter to prevent laser emission until a desired time, a method of producing short laser pulses at high energy
Spot Size	diameter of the focal point
TEM	Transverse electomagnetic mode
TEM/oo	a bell shaped distribution of light energy across the laser beam cross section
Thermal Effect	the influence of heating on surrounding tissue
Tunable Laser	a system that can be tuned to emit laser light over a continuous range of wavelengths and frequencies
Vaporization	conversion of a solid or liquid into a vapor
Watt	unit of power equivalent to one joule per second

INFORMATION FOR PATIENTS

DERMATOLOGY VASCULAR TUMORS

Pre-Operative Information

What to Do to Prepare for Laser Surgery?
1. Arrive at the Outpatient Department.
   a. Necessary forms will need to be signed.
   b. You will need to verify your medical insurance.
2. What <u>to do</u> the day of you Laser Surgery.
   a. Have a responsible adult accompany you, to take you home after your procedure.
   b. Wear comfortable, casual clothes.
   c. Wear no make-up.
   d. Tell us if you have any ALLERGIES to food or drugs.
   e. Tell the doctor or nurse what medications you are taking.
3. What you <u>should not do</u> the day of Surgery.
   a. Leave your valuables or extra money at home.
   b. <u>Do not eat or drink</u> after midnight, unless you receive other instructions.

Why Is Laser Being Used on My Surgery?
1. A laser is an intense, straight beam of light on one pure color that has intense energy.
2. The laser can cut like a knife, coagulate small blood vessels, decreasing blood loss, or vaporize tissue into harmless vapor.
3. The laser beam can be beamed down quartz fibers and into a tube that can be passed into a body cavity connected to a lens that the doctor can look through, and destroy tumors or other tissue in the body cavity.
4. The laser is so precise that it does less damages to other tissue and that decreases the swelling that may occur, and promotes quicker healing.
5. Laser Surgery is not as painful, although pain is subjective, however, patients have expressed less post operative discomfort after laser procedures.

What to Expect During the Laser Procedure.

1. The procedure will be done under local anesthesia (like in a dentist office), so there will be an injection with a very small needle, that causes the area to be numb.
2. There will be a smell as the laser interacts with the tissue and the sound of a suction machine taking away the "smoke."
3. There will be special glasses that you will need to wear during the procedure, that protects your eyes from the laser beam.
4. If the procedure hurts, tell the physician right away.

What to Expect After Laser Treatment?

The following information explains what happens to your skin after the laser procedure:

1. Immediately, after the laser procedure on your skin it will turn white.
2. After a few days the treated areas will form crusts.
3. After the crust falls off the laser treated areas will look red, this will be expected.
4. The areas will gradually become lighter in color within the next few weeks and months.

How to Care for theLaser Treated Area

1. Wash the area gently with mild soap and warm water and rinse well.
2. Gently pat the area dry and apply a thin layer of ointment (pre scribed by the physician) over the area.
3. Do not cover unless the area is irritated by clothing.
4. Continue the above treatment until the crust has fallen off.
5. If you are a women, apply make up lightly on treated areas only after the scab has fallen off.

What to Avoid After Laser Treatments?

1. Avoid swimming until the treated area is completely healed.
2. Treated skin may be overly sensitive to sun and always use #15 sunscreen, when out in the sun.
3. Continue to use a skin softening agent prescribed by physician.

Information for Patients

Followup Appointment:

DATE: _____

PHYSICIAN _____ M.D.

_____   _____ R.N.
   Signature of Patient   Signature of Nurse

HOME CARE INSTRUCTIONS
LASER TREATMENTS

____Cervical Intraepithelial Neoplasia (CIN)   ____Vaginal Warts
____Condyloma   ____Herpes
____Vulvar lesions   ____VIN

The following instructions are to help you care for yourself when you return home, these are guidelines for your post laser procedure.

MEDICATIONS
- ____ No medications, including non-prescription, unless ordered by the surgeon, for 24 hours.
- ____ Resume your own medications.

WOUND CARE AND HYGIENE
- ____ Wash in warm tub of water or "ocean" water, twice a day to relieve discomfort. Pat dry with towel or hair dryer.
- ____ No intercourse until
  Apply,_____to lesions, cover with a sterile gauze pad or sanitary napkin. **Wash hands** before touching the lesions.
- ____ No Tampons or douching until_____

ACTIVITY
- ____ Resume normal activities on_____
- ____ Return to work /school

ANESTHESIA PRECAUTIONS
- ____ No special precautions
- ____ Do Not operate a motor vehicle, power tools, or make important decisions for 24 hours.
- ____ Do not drink alcoholic beverages for 24 hours.
- ____ Arrange for an adult to remain with you for 24 hours.

Information for Patients

EXPECTATIONS _____ Drainage from lesions.
AFTER SURGERY _____ Minimal pain, take _____, as
                                      need for discomfort.
                        _____ Mild burning sensation at operative site.

CALL YOUR DOCTOR
                        _____ Excessive red bleeding.
                        _____ Temperature above 100°
                        _____ Excessive vaginal bleeding
                        _____ If unable to contact doctor, go to the **Emergency Room.**

ADDITIONAL INSTRUCTIONS _____
_____
_____

Your Doctor's Appointment is on _____

Physician's Signature: _____

Patient's/Guardian Signature: _____

Nurse's Signature: _____

JOB DESCRIPTION

TITLE: LASER PROGRAM COORDINATOR

DEPARTMENT: LASER CENTER

General Summary:

The Laser Program Coordinator administers the program. Directs the program development and assists in the education assessment of physicians and nurses to plan the education programs. Coordinates the Public Relations components of the laser program. Defines the physician referral system for the facility with methods to analyze these trends. Implements the statistical reporting system to hospital administration.The Laser Program Coordinator reports to the Vice President of Operations.

Principle Duties and Responsibilities

A. Works intra-departmentally ,with each administrator to coordinate all laser activity that is integrated in their department to assure ongoing development of the laser program.

B. Work with the appropriate departments or committee's to integrate the laser program into the hospital's Quality Assurance, Risk Management and Nursing Practice Committee to plan quality patient care.

C. Continue to assess and plan laser education programs for physician and nursing staff on a continuum.

D. Monitor's laser usage to assure there is NO conflict in scheduling laser systems and accessories, inter-departmentally , where the lasers are being used.

E. Continue to refine and delineate hospital and nursing policies, to include safety polices and procedures for the laser program.

Patient Care

A. Directs the Clinical Nurse's activities related to patients having laser procedures, to include assessment, planning, implementation, and evaluation.

B. Directs the Bio-Laser Technicians activity to assure that all laser systems and accessories or available and functional for each laser procedure.

Job Description

C. Evaluates patient care by reviewing the post-operative assessment process with the Clinical Nurse to assure optimum patient care.

D. Establishes a collaborative practice approach with the physicians using the laser to enhance their practice and assure quality patient care.

Fiscal Management:

A. Develop and maintains methods to effectively control costs both fiscal expenses and human resources for the laser program.

B. Develops and manages the operational budget for the laser center, and is able to justify any variances that occur.

C. Works inter-departmentally to maintain a standard inventory of disposable items used for laser procedures to be cost effective.

D. Maintains documents of all transactions to assist in the planning of both human resource, expense and capital budgets.

Facilities Management:

A. Assures all safety policies and procedures have been approved and are followed and any variances reported to the appropriate committees.

B. Directs the Bio-Laser Technicians activities to assure maintenance of all laser equipment and accessories, making sure that they are functional at all times.

Personnnel Supervision:

A. Has responsibility for the orientation to the laser program all other employee's of the laser center.

B. Directs the nursing and bio-medical activities of the laser program and makes a daily assessment as to the progress of care administered to the laser patients.

C. Evaluates the employee's work performance in a fair and expedient manner, offering feedback and counseling to maximize their productivity.

D. Promotes a positive work atmosphere to enhance the employee opportunity for productivity.

E. Is acquainted with each employee's activities to understand and intervene or assumed those activities as needed.

Qualifications:

A. Graduate from a recognized college with a degree in Business or Hospital Administration or school of nursing with current license of the state.
B. Three or more years of successful experience as an administrator or program manager in the health care field.
C. Experience is a surgical environment desired by not required.
D. Other experiences helpful are:
    1. Budget development and management.
    2. Laser education.
    3. Public speaking or related public relations experience.
    4. Knowledge of community resources.
    5. Verbal and written communication skills.
    6. Ability to be a self-directed person.

Appendix

Approval:

The above statements are intended to describe the general nature and level of the work being performed by the person assigned to this job classification. They are not intended to be construed as an exhaustive list of all responsibilities, duties and skills required of the job classification.

TITLE: **LASER PROGRAM COORDINATOR**

APPROVED BY:
ADMINISTRATION:_____
                    Name   Date

HUMAN RESOURCES: _____
                    Name   Date

EMPLOYEE SIGNATURE:_____

Revised: _____Date

Suggested Content Outline for Orienting Nurse to Lasers

1. Laser Bio-Physics
2. Tissue Effects of Different Lasers
3. Types of Surgical Lasers
4. Safety Procedures for Each Laser System

    a. Patient and Protection
        1.) Eye Wear
        2.) Viewing Windows
        3.) Matte' Instruments

    b. Evironmental Protection
        1.) Warning Signs
        2.) Drapes
        3.) Smoke Evacuators

    C. Electrical Safety
        1.) Power outlet interfaces
        2.) Water connecting systems

    D. Laser Start-up and Shut-down Procedures

    E. Special Procedures
        1.) Anesthestic gases
        2.) High Oxygen environments

5. Fiber maintainence
6. Nursing Interventions during laser procedures.
7. Patient Education
8. Policies and Procedures
9. F.D.A. Regulations and Informed Consent
10. Optional Content for Nurse Managers
    a. Organizational Structure
    b. Laser Acquisitions
    c. DRG's and charging mechanisms
    d. Space Planning
    e. Staffing Assignments
    f. Budget preparation
11. Laser Demonstrations with return demonstrations.

HOSPITAL REIMBURSEMENT INFORMATION
ESOPHAGEAL CANCER
LASER ABLATION

Admission date: _____ Time: _____ Orgin: _____
Discharge date: _____ Time: _____ Payor code: ___
Patient Birthdate: _____ Sex ___ F ___ M
Social Security Number: _____ Length of Stay: ___
Admission type: _____ Admission Service: _____
Admission Source: _____ Dicharge Service: _____
Disposition: _____
Principal Diagnosis: 151.0 Malignant Neoplasm Stomach, Cardia.
Principal Procedure: 42.39 Destruction, Esophageal Lesion, Date:
Other Procedure: 42.23 Esophagoscopy   ,   Date:

D.R.G.: 155 P Stomach, Esophageal & Doudenal Procedures Age: 18-69 W/O CC

M.D.C. 06   Dieseases & Disorders of the Digestive System

Relative Weight: _____
Mean Lenght of Stay: 13.0   Outlier Cutoff: 35
Principal Diagnosis: 151.0   Mal. Neo. Stomach, Cardia
Procedure Code Used: 42.39   Destruction Esophageal Les.
Any Diagnosis Used: _____
C.C. Diagnosis Used: _____
Coded: _____ Id.# _____
Assembled: _____ Id.# _____
Expected Reimbursement: $11,300.00

I Certify that the narrative description of the principal and secodary diagnoses and the major procedures performed are accurate and complete to the best of my knowledge.

_____   _____ M.D.
Date   Attending Physician Signature

Classroom Requirements for Laser Workshops

1. CLASSROOM IN A CONVENIENT LOCATION, SET UP IN CLASSROOM STYLE.
2. AUDIO-VISUAL NEEDS:
   a. 2 - 35 mm slide projector with 4 extra carousals, make sure there is an extra bulb and an extension on the "clicker"
   b. 3/4 inch video player and monitor
   c. 1/2 inch VHS video player and monitor
   d. projection screen
   e. pointer
   f. blackboard or flip chart with chalk or markers
3. A TELEPHONE NEAR BY WITH EXTENSION NUMBER POSTED.
4. TELEPHONE OPERATORS AND SECURITY NOTIFIED WHEN AND WHERE THE LASER PROGRAMS ARE BEING HELD.
5. DIETARY NEEDS:
   a. PHYSICIAN COURSES: **(FOR EACH COURSE DATE)**
      1.) Continental Breakfast with; coffee, tea, juice, danish and fruit.
      2.) Fill coffee and tea pots at break usually 10:00 am.
      3.) Lunch provided to included: cold buffet with salad, sandwiches, dessert, drinks to include soda.
      4.) Afternoon break; soda, coffee and cookies.
      5.) **FRIDAY EVENING PHYSICS COURSES AT 6:00 pm;** light refreshment; coffee, tea, soda, cheese and crackers and fruit.
   b. NURSES COURSES: **(FOR EACH COURSE DATE)**
      1. **FRIDAY EVENING AT 6:00 pm;** light refreshment; coffee, tea, soda, cheese and crackers and fruit.

2.) Continental Breakfast with; coffee, tea, juice, danish and fruit.
3.) Fill coffee and tea pots at break usually 10:00 am.
4.) Lunch provided to included: cold buffet with salad, sandwiches, dessert, drinks to include soda.
5.) Afternoon break; soda, coffee and cookies.
6. HAVE **"LASER WORKSHOP"** SIGNS MADE WITH ARROWS INDICATING THE DIRECTION OF THE WORK SHOP THAT CAN BE POSTED.

SELECTED READING

1. Murphy, Ellen, R.N.,MSN,J.D.,
   Legal Implications of the O.R. Laser Use.
   Today's O.R. Nurse, June 6 (6): 32, 1984.

2. Fay, M.F. R.N.
   Harnessing Light For Lasers,
   Todays O.R. Nurse, May (5): 8-11, 1984

3. Baroiko, A.A.,
   "A Spendid Light" Lasers
   National Geographic 165 (3), 1984

4. Huether, Sue, Phd,
   How Lasers Work
   AORN J 38 (2): 217-22, 1983

5. Lundergan, D, et. al.
   Nurses Administrative Responsibilities
   for Lasers
   AORN J 38 (2): 217-22, 1983

6. Casey, K.R. et. al.,
   Intratracheal Fire Ignited By The Nd: YAG
   Laser, During Treatment of Tracheal
   Stenosis
   Chest 84 (3): 295-6, 1983

7. Dixon, J.A. M.D.
   Surgical Implications of Lasers
   AORN J 38 (2): 223-30, 1983

8. Cayton M.M., R.N.
   Nursing Responsibilities in Laser Surgery
   Medical Instrumentation
   7 (6): 410-21, 1983

9. Perrin Ed.
   Laser Therapy for Diabetic Retinopathy
   American Journal of Nursing
   80:664-5, 1980

10. Mylotte M. et. al.,
    Beaming in on Women...
    Laser use in Modern Gynecologic Practice
    Nursing Mirror 9 (149) 26-8, 1979

11. Witty K.T.
    Eye Care for Your Diabetic Patients
    Patients Care 2: 174-6, 1978

Selected Reading

12. Zadeh, A.T.,M.D., Kirchner, Beverly, R.N.
    Outpatient Hemorrhoidectomy
    Laser Treatment and Case Results
    AORN J December 1986, Vol. 44 No. 6

13. Martin, Catherine, R.N., B.S.,
    Olson, Elizebeth, M.S. R.N.,
    Photodynamic Laser Surgery
    Today's O.R. Nurse Vol. 7, N0. 10, 1985

14. Sakallaris, Bonnie, R.N., M.S.N.,
    Laser Therapy for Cardiovascular Disease
    Heart and Lung, The Journal of Critical Care
    September, 1987, Vol. 16, No. 5.

15. Gervaize, Patricia A., Phd,
    Beresford, James, M.B. ChB.
    Outpatient Gynecological Laser Therapy
    Canadian Operating Room Nursing Journal
    October 1984, p.p. 34-42

16. Mc Caughan, James, M.D.,
    Laser in Medicine and Surgery:
    Introduction
    Internal Medicine
    March 1984, Vol 5, No. 3.

17. Mackety, Carolyn J. R.N. M.A.,
    The Laser Committee:
    Its Role in Quality Assurance
    Health Care Strategic Management
    August 1984, p.p.13-16.

18. Risk Analysis: Laser Use and Safety
    ECRI
    January 1984

19. Larrow, L, R.N., Noe, J. M.D.,
    PortWine Stain Hemangiomas
    American Journal of Nursing
    May, 1982, Pgs. 786-790

20. Snow, J.C., Norton, M. L.,
    Laser and Anesthesia
    American of Nurse Anesthetists Journal
    July 192, pgs. 7-11.

LASER LOG

PATIENT NAME: MEDICAL RECORD #: PHYSICIAN: DATE OF BIRTH: PHONE #	ADDRESSOGRAPH

DATE: ___/___/___/ DOSA_____ S.U._____ I.P._____ DRG_____ CODE_____
PRE-OPERATIVE DIAGNOSIS:_____
OPERATIVE PROCEDURE:_____
ANESTHESIA: GENERAL____LOCAL____SPINAL____SEDATION____NONE_____
ANESTHESOLOGY STAFF: ATTENDING_____M.D. RESIDENT_____M..D.
CRNA_____R.N. SUPERVISOR_____M.D. LASER E.T._____ USED:

TYPE OF LASER USED: CO/2____C.W. ND: YAG_____ARGON____ND: YAG EYE_____
EYE PROTECTION ON PATIENT_____STAFF_____SIGNS UP: YES_____NO_____
WINDOWS COVERED: YES____NO____ENDOSCOPE: YES____NO____TYPE:_____
MICROSCOPE: YES____NO_____ LENS: 200_____250_____300_____400_____
EYE LENS: YAG ABRAHAM_____CAPSULOTOMY____IRRIDECTONY____PYEMEN_____
    TROKEL____ARGON GOLDMAN____RODENSTOCK____ABRAHAM____RITCH_____

LASER ON AT:_____OFF AT:_____E. PLS_____J CUM E._____J

RATE	MODE	WATTS	TIME

FIBER CLAIBRATION_____% TYPE OF TIP_____
TYPE OF HAND PIECE:_____ TYPE OF FIBER:_____

NOTES

NOTES

NOTES

NOTES

NOTES